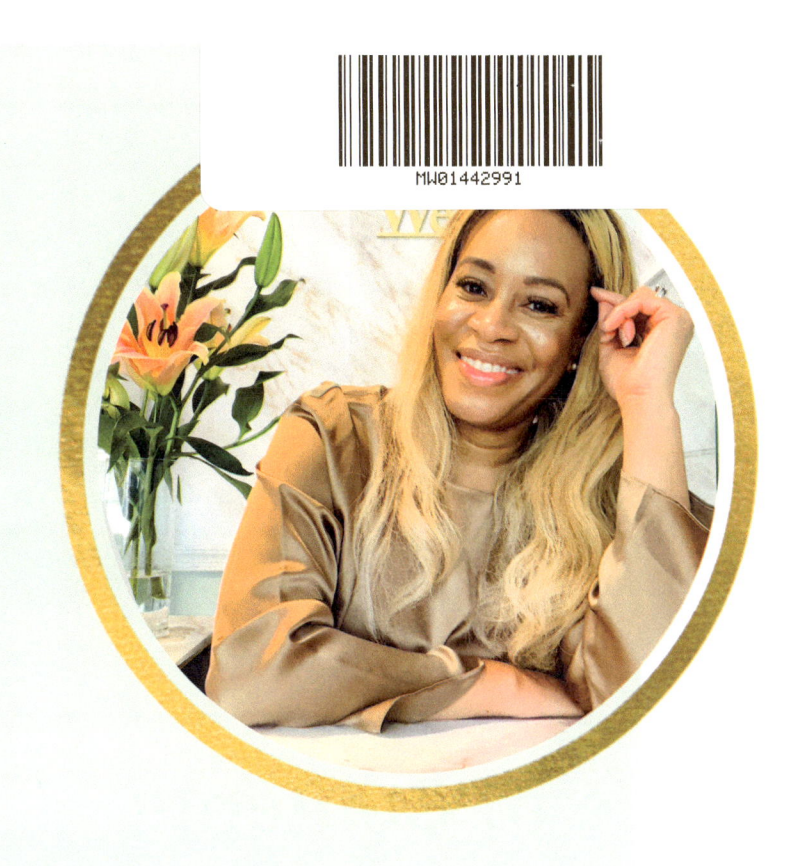

Welcome to Beautifully Well in 30 Days!

The secret sauce to sustainable weight loss success is the following:

1. Accepting where you are.
2. Willingness to start small.
3. Tracking food and activity.

This program is designed to make healthy motivating, and of course fun! Name your journey and hop into the digital wellness suite to make your goals an achievable reality.

Nik Sweeney,
National Board Certified Health & Wellness Coach

Digital Access Online Program

This document contains materials for the PreventT2 Curriculum and the Beautifully Well Lifestyle Program.

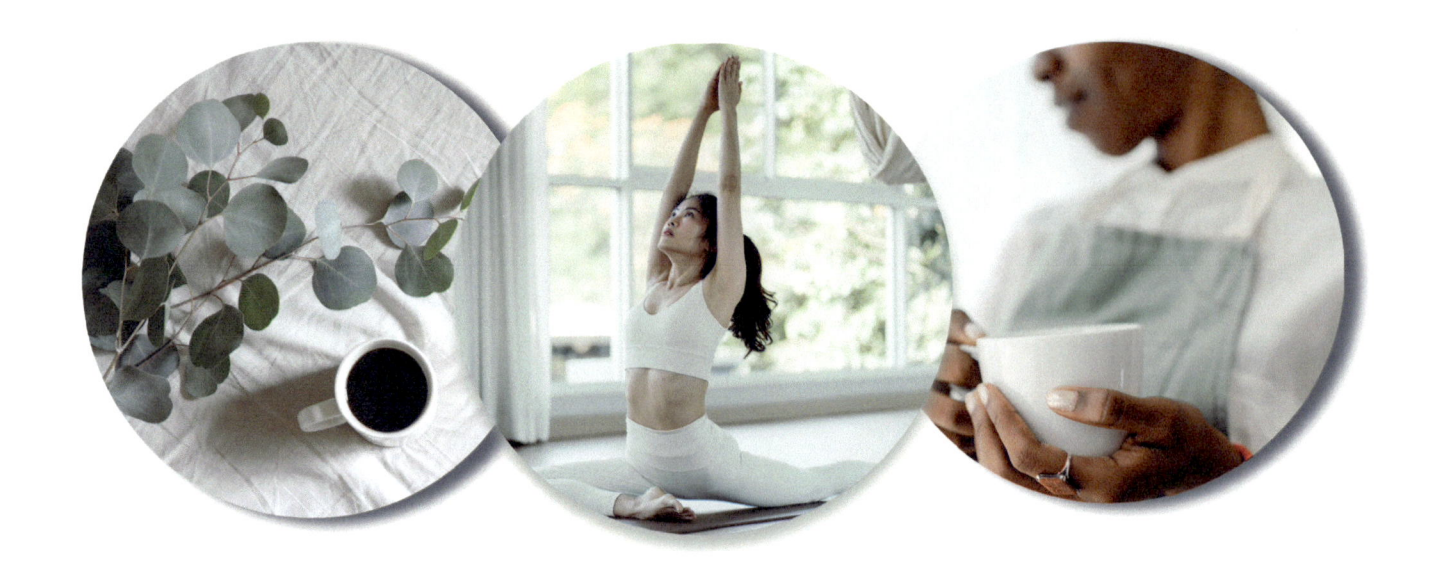

Table of Contents

Prevention. 1
Heart Challenge 2
Stress Management 3
Mindful Eating 9
Embrace Movement 15
Weekly Plans 20
Vision Board 22
Bonus: Weight Management Meal Plan 33

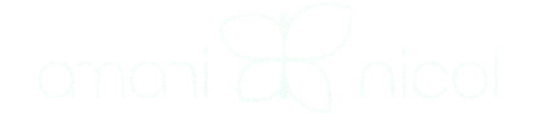

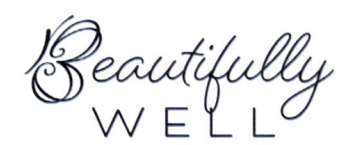

Prevention

Prediabetes

Prediabetes means that your blood sugar is higher than normal. But it's not high enough for type 2 diabetes.
- More than 1 in 3 American adults has prediabetes.
- 9 out of 10 people with prediabetes don't know they have it.

	Fasting blood sugar level (mg/dl)	**Hemoglobin A1C%**
Normal	Less than 100	Less than 5.7
Pre-diabetes	100-125	5.7 to less than 6.5
Diabetes	126 and higher	6.5 and above

If you have prediabetes, you are more likely to get:
- Diabetes
- Heart disease
- Stroke

The good news is that losing weight and being active can cut your risk of type 2 diabetes in half.

- One goal of this program is to lose at least 5 to 7 percent of your starting weight in the next six months. For instance, if you weigh 200 pounds, you will lose 10 to 14 pounds.
- Multiply your weight by the percentage you want to lose (5%, 6%, or 7%).

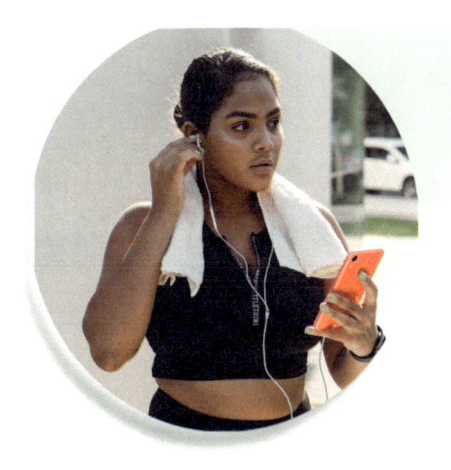

Activity Goal
At least 150 minutes of activity each week at a moderate pace or more.

Weight Goal
I weigh _____ pounds.

In the next six months, I will:

Lose at least _____ (5/6/7) % of my body weight

Lose at least _____ pounds

Reach _____ pounds

Source: American College of Sports Medicine (https://www.acsm.org/docs/brochures/reducing-s edentary-behaviors-sitting-less-and-mov- ing-more.pdf) and Heart Foundation (https://heartfoundation.org.au/images/uploads/publications/PA-Sitting-Less-Adults.pdf)

Seven Day Heart Challenge

Try these tips for keeping track of your blood pressure at home:

- Always take your blood pressure at the same time every day for 7 days.
- Take at least two readings, 1 or 2 minutes apart.
- Click the QR code below to learn how to correctly measure your blood pressure.

American College of Cardiology and AHA 2017 Guidelines on blood pressure levels

	Normal	Elevated	Hypertension
Systolic	<120	120-129	> 130
Diastolic	< 80	< 80	> 80

Date	Morning			Evening		
	Time of reading	Reading 1	Reading 2	Time of reading	Reading 1	Reading 2
Sept. 1, 2022	8 a.m.	139/82	141/82	6 p.m.	145/85	142/83

Nurse Tiffany demonstrates the proper way to measure your blood pressure in this video.

Stress Management

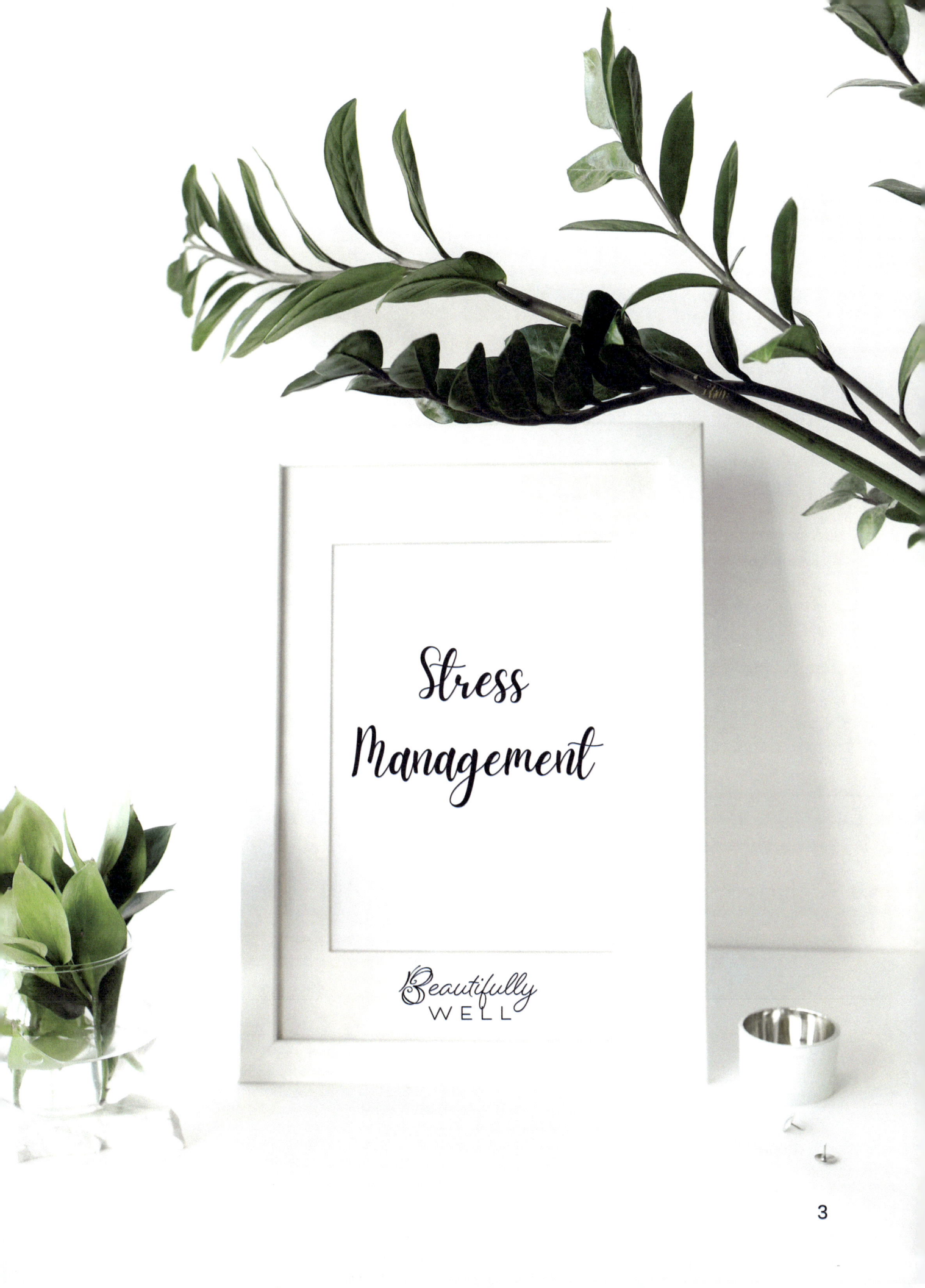

Beautifully WELL

Stressed out Rachael....

Rachael is 45 years old. She feels pulled in all directions. Her children are still in high school. Her father has bad health problems. Plus, Rachael works full time and is divorced.

Rachael's doctor tells her she's at risk for type 2 diabetes. He urges her to lose weight by eating well and getting active.

For Rachael, caring for herself is just one more thing on her to-do list.

After her doctor's visit, Rachael goes home and eats a lot of ice cream to feel better.

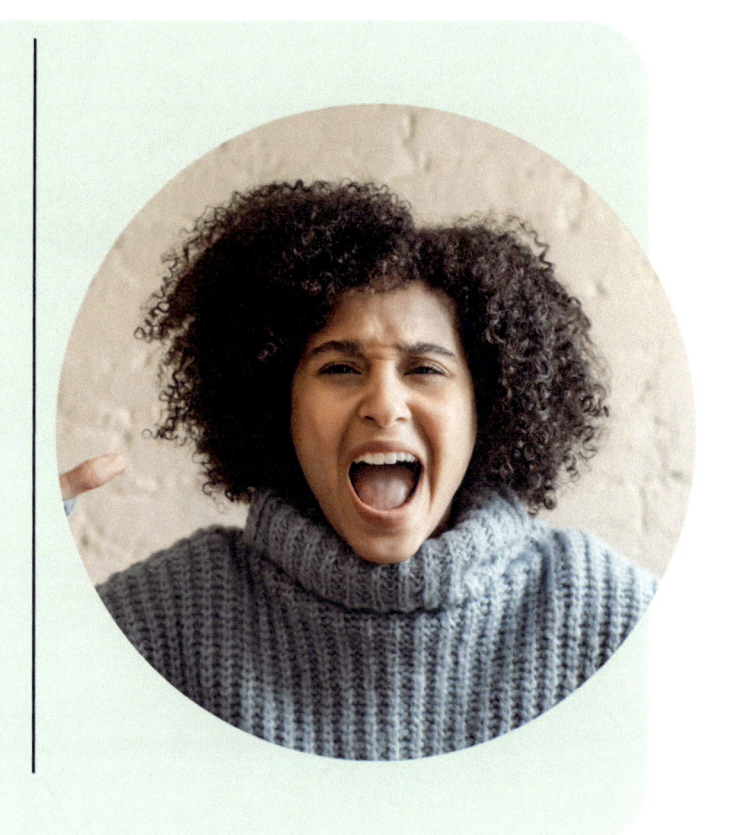

By the end of the day when her children are in bed and her dad is content, Rachael turns on her favorite tv show, grabs her bottle of wine and bowl of ice cream.

Her nightly routine feels good for the moment, but she knows her health will not improve if she continues to neglect her health.

What would you do if you were in her shoes? The answer is not drink more wine.

When you feel stressed, you may:
- Drink too much alcohol ● Forget things
- Putting off things you need to do
- Unproductive days ● Sleep too little and or too much ● Smoke ● Take too much medicine

You may also:
- Making unhealthy choices ● Slack off on fitness goals ● Spend too much time watching TV or videos or using the computer

When you feel stressed, you may feel:
- Angry ● Annoyed ● Anxious
- Confused ● Impatient ● Sad ● Worried

You may also have:
- Aching head, back, or neck
- Racing heart-beat ● Tight muscles
- Upset stomach

Ways to Reduce Stress

There's no surefire way to prevent stress. But there are ways to make your life less stressful. Try these tips.

- **Ask for help.** Friends and family care about you and want the best for you.
- **Be tidy.** Keep your things in order.
- **Get enough sleep.** Shoot for 7- 8 hours per night.
- **Have fun!** Walk with a friend, read a book, … whatever makes you happy.
- **Just say "no."** Learn how to say no to things you don't want or need to do.
- **Know yourself.** Know your stressors and plan how to cope with them.
- **Make a to-do list.** Put the most important things on top.
- **Remind yourself.** Use notes, calendars, timers— whatever works for you.
- **Set small, doable goals.** Divide large goals into smaller chunks.
  - **Solve problems.** Solve problems promptly so they don't become a source of stress.
- **Take care of your body and mind.** Know when its time to take a pause.

Feeling stressed? Put down the cookies! Instead, try these healthy ways to cope with stress.

- **Count to 20 in your head.** This can give your brain a needed break.
  - **Soothe yourself.** Get a massage, take a hot bath, have a cup of herbal tea, or put on some calming music.
  - **Give yourself a pep talk.** Say something calming, like: "There's no rush. I can take my time."
- **Try some new ways to relax.** You'll find them on the next page.
- **Stretch.** Find your favorite stretch routine.

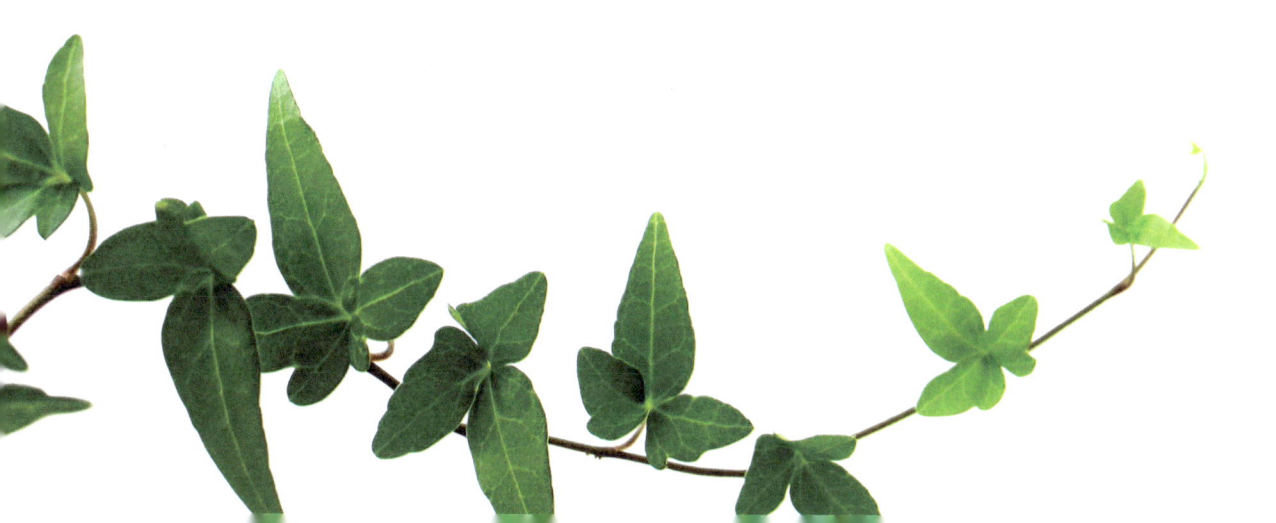

Ways to Reduce Stress

Take a breather. If you can, take a break from whatever is making you feel stressed.

- **Talk about your feelings.** Tell a friend or counselor how you feel.
- **Cut back on caffeine.** Caffeine can make you feel jumpy and anxious.
- **Get moving!** Do something active—even if it's just a walk around the block.
- **Do something fun.** Go out dancing, go shopping, call a friend. Do whatever you enjoy—as long as it's healthy.
- **Think clearly.** Things may not be as bad as they seem to be.

A quick tip when you are feeling overwhelmed but feeling tempted to put more on your plate. Think about your mental capacity and not the time on your watch. Your watch could indicate you have the time to do the last minute task or favor, but your mind and body says no.

It's ok to say no. When you say no, you empower others to figure it out. And guess what, they will.

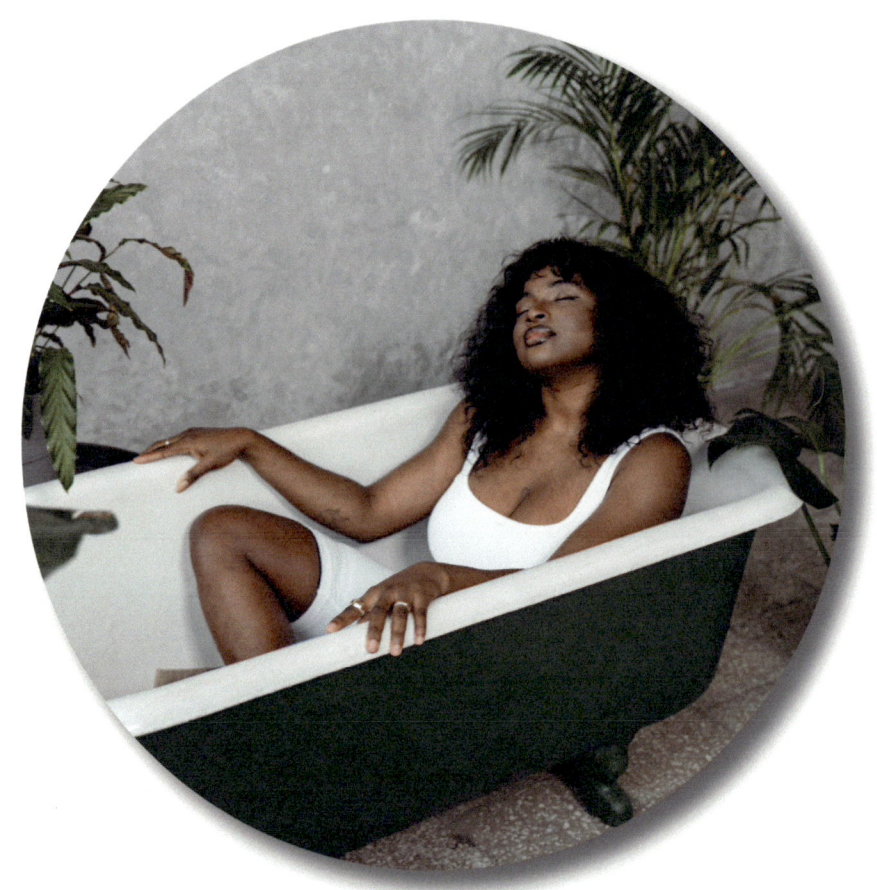

How Will You Reduce Stress in Your Life?

_____
_____
_____
_____
_____
_____
_____
_____
_____
_____

Self-Care CHECKLIST

Self-care is an intentional act honoring your need to pause and make time for you.

Physical Self-Care	M	T	W	T	F	S	S
Cook a healthy, nourishing meal							
Schedule a doctors appointment							
Exercise or move your body							
Follow a skincare routine							
Take a long bath or shower							

Mind & Soul Self-Care	M	T	W	T	F	S	S
Attend a workshop or class							
Read for 30 minutes							
Listen to a podcast episode							
Learn something new							
Plan out your week in advance							

Emotional Self-Care	M	T	W	T	F	S	S
Practice daily gratitude							
Spend time with a loved one							
Foster a positive mindset							
Spend time outdoors and in nature							
Journal your thoughts							

Mindful Eating

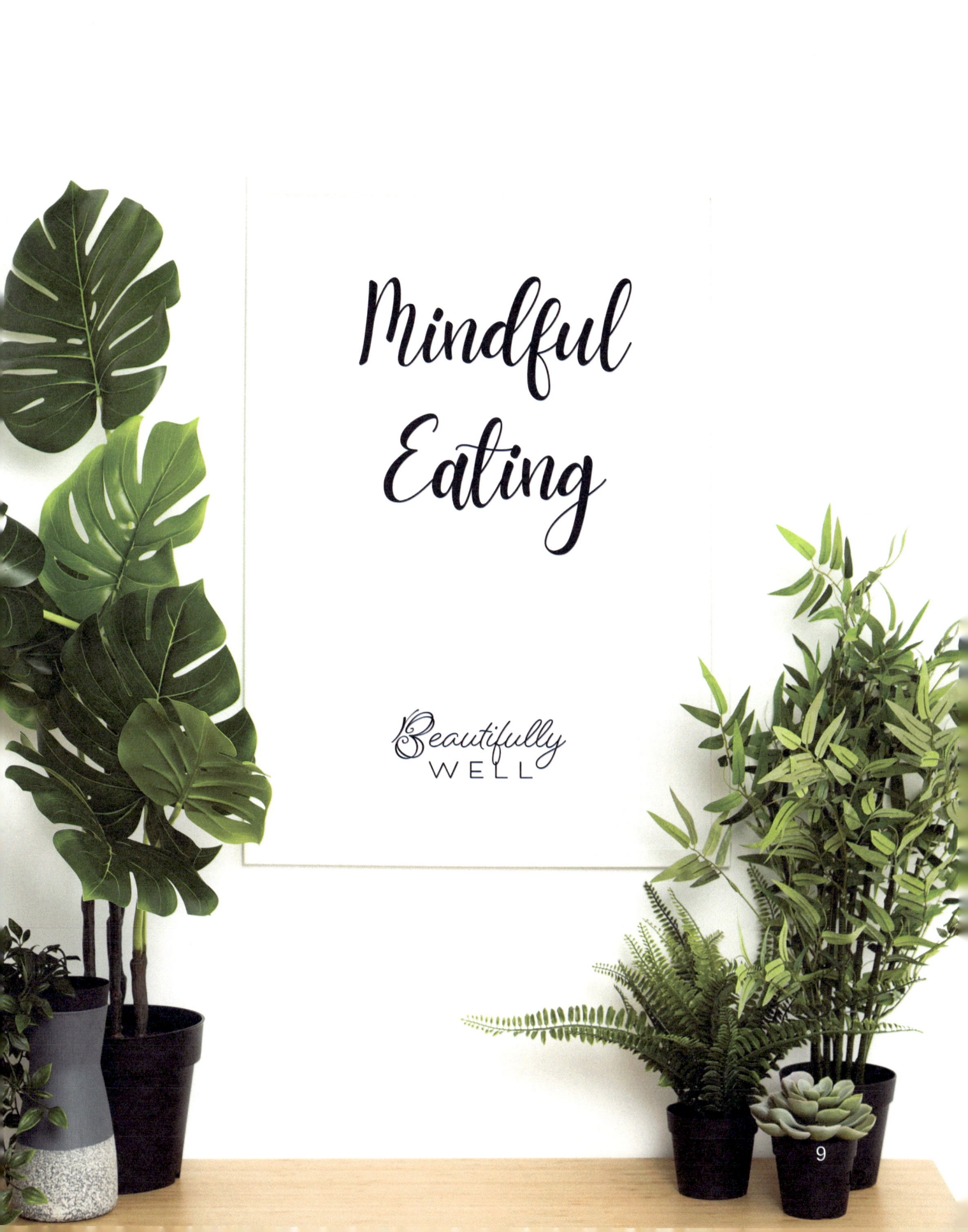

Beautifully WELL

Calorie-Counting Patti.....

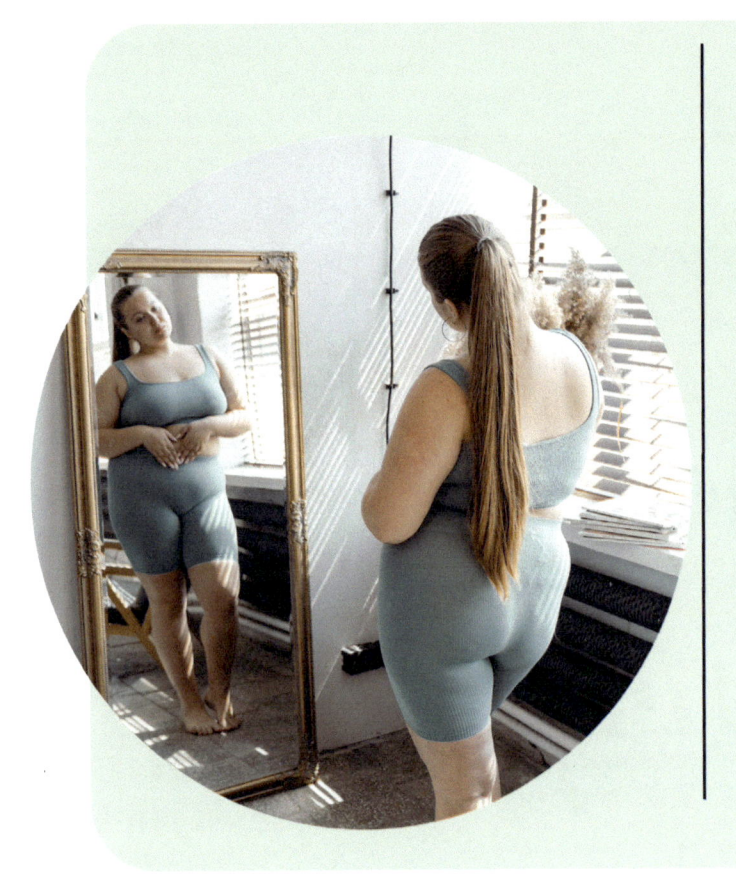

Patti: 47 years old - 240 pounds.

At risk for type 2 diabetes.

Doctor urges her to lose 40 pounds at (1 lb / week).

A healthy gradual loss of 1 to 2 pounds a week is sustainable for most adults. To lose 1 pound a week, she needs to burn 3,500 more calories than she takes in each week or 500 calories per day.

Ways that Patti could burn 500 more calories than she consumes

1. Eat 500 fewer calories per day.
2. Being more active.
3. Cut 500 calories per day through a mix of eating and activity.

Patti needs about 2,200 calories a day to function and maintain the same weight. If she cuts 500 calories per day, she's left with 1,700 calories.

Let's start with the calories she takes in, then we'll subtract the calories she burns:

2,000 – 310 = 1,690

Patti beats her goal by 10 calories!

These days, Patti is losing about 1 pound each week through a mixture of eating and activity. And she's halfway to her goal weight.

Patti's Sunday routine:

- She eats a 400-calorie breakfast.
- Takes a brisk walk burning 90 calories.
- She has a 200-calorie mid-morning snack.
- She enjoys a 500-calorie lunch.
- She has a 100-calorie afternoon snack.
- She mows the lawn and burns 100 calories.
- She has a 600-calorie dinner.
- Then, she takes a longer brisk
- walk and burns 120 calories.
- She has a 200-calorie bedtime
- snack.

Nutrition Tip

Create a healthy meal by listing items that you like.

Non-Starchy Vegetables
• Asparagus • Broccoli • Cabbage • Carrots • Celery • Cucumbers • Leafy greens • Mushrooms • Onions • Peppers • Tomatoes

Grains and Starchy Foods:
• 100% corn tortillas • Whole grain cereal & bread • Black beans • Brown rice • Corn • Green peas • Lentils • Oatmeal • Popcorn • Potatoes • Yams

Fruit:
• Apples • Apricots • Blueberries • Dates • Grapefruit • Grapes • Oranges • Strawberries

Protein Foods:
• Eggs (but limit yolks) • Fish and seafood (catfish, cod, shrimp) • Lean meat (ground beef, chicken and turkey without skin, pork loin) • Nuts (limit due to high fat)

Dairy Foods:
• Low-fat cheese • Plain soy or almond milk • Plain nonfat or low-fat yogurt • Skim or low-fat milk

Drinks
• Coffee without sugar • Sparking Water • Tea without sugar • Water

You'll want to make:

- 1/2 of plate non-starchy veggies (i.e. broccoli, lettuce, peppers)
- 1/4 of your plate grains and starchy foods (such as potatoes, oatmeal)
- 1/4 of your plate protein foods (such as chicken, lean meat, fish)

What are YOUR calorie needs?

Your daily calorie needs are the calories you need to maintain your weight. This number is based on your age, sex, height, build, and weight. It doesn't take your activity level into account.

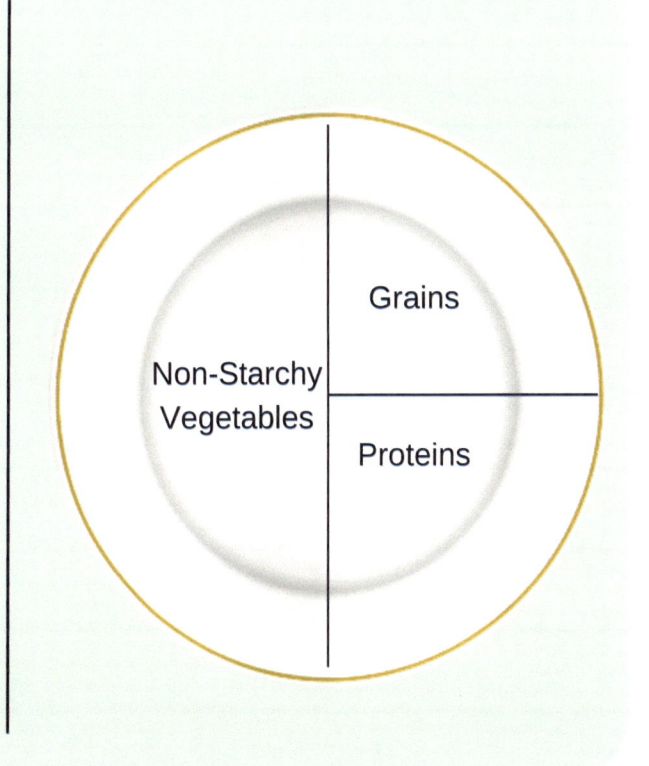

Track Your Food

Try to track your food each day. Start by tracking what and when you eat. When you get comfortable with this, you can start tracking how much you eat, and then calories.

Ways to find out how much you eat:

- Measuring cups and spoons
- Kitchen scale
- Food labels
- Calculator

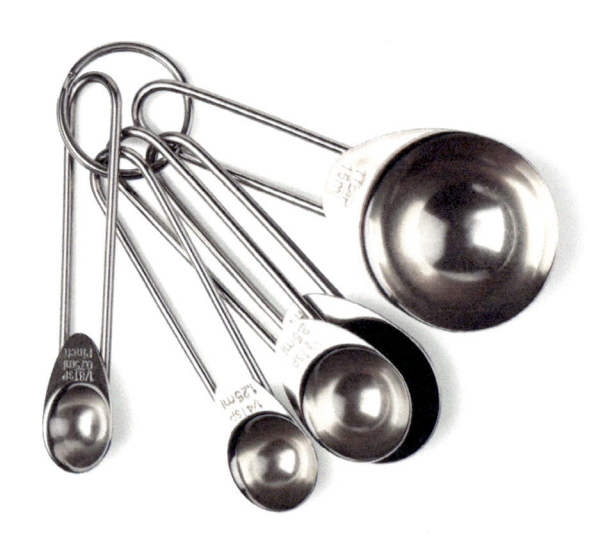

Options for food tracking:

Fitbit

Apple Watch

Spiral notebook

Smart phone apps

Computer apps

Voice recording

Photo of your food

*Digital Food Journals are available in the online program.

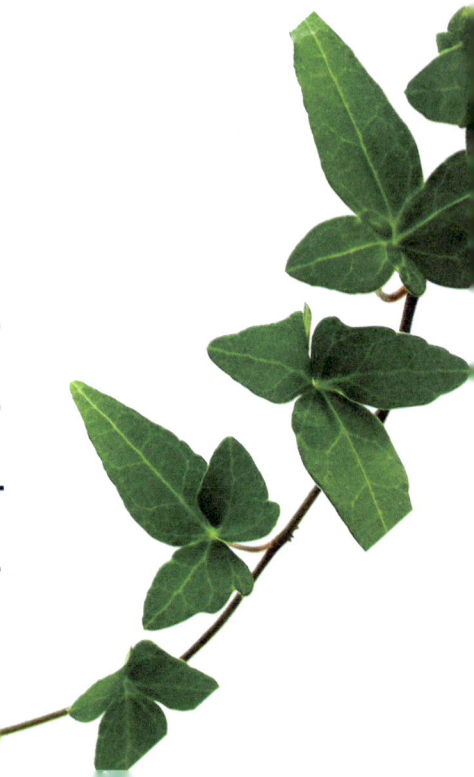

Your Common Challenges

Challenges:

_____

_____

_____

Ways to Cope:

_____

_____

_____

_____

Become a Food Label Master

1. Serving Size

Notice the number of servings. All the other facts on the label are based on this amount. If you eat the whole package, multiply all the other facts on the label by two.

2. Calories

Calories are the amount of energy you get from a serving of this food. Many Americans eat more calories than needed. Try to get less than 30% of your calories from fat.

3. Limit These Nutrients

Eating too much fat, saturated fat, trans fat, cholesterol, or sodium can raise your risk of certain health problems. These include heart disease, some cancers, and high blood pressure.

4. Get Enough of These Nutrients

Fiber, vitamin A, vitamin C, calcium, and iron: Eating enough of these nutrients can improve your health and lower your risk of certain health problems.

For instance, getting enough calcium can help strengthen your bones and teeth. Eating plenty of fiber can help you lose weight and lower your cholesterol.

Nutrition Facts

8 servings per container
Serving size 2/3 cup (55g)

Amount per serving
Calories 230

	% Daily Value*
Total Fat 8g	10%
Saturated Fat 1g	5%
Trans Fat 0g	
Cholesterol 0mg	0%
Sodium 160mg	7%
Total Carbohydrate 37g	13%
Dietary Fiber 4g	14%
Total Sugars 12g	
Includes 10g Added Sugars	20%
Protein 3g	
Vitamin D 2mcg	10%
Calcium 260mg	20%
Iron 8mg	45%
Potassium 235mg	6%

* The % Daily Value (DV) tells you how much a nutrient in a serving of food contributes to a daily diet. 2,000 calories a day is used for general nutrition advice.

*The digital food journal available to you in this program has a national nutrition database that can be used to get nutrition facts.

Ways to Eat Fewer Calories

Here are some ways to cut calories at each meal. Try these healthy swaps.

Breakfast Swaps

Cereal with 2% or whole milk.

Scrambled eggs in butter

Top your cereal with low-fat or fat-free milk.

Use a non-stick pan and cooking spray

Lunch Swaps

Extra meat added to sandwich

French fries paired with sandwich

Cream or meat-based soups Dressing poured on salads

French fries or chips for a side dish

Add extra veggies like cucumber, lettuce, tomato and onion

Pair fruit with sandwich

Vegetable-based broth soups

Salad as a side dish

Dinner Swaps

Vegetable fried in butter or oil

Ground meat throughout lasagna

Vegetables steamed or grilled, flavored with lemon juice and herbs.

Shredded vegetable substituted for some ground meat

Snack Swaps

Oil popped popcorn or oil roasted nuts.

Vending machine package of peanut butter crackers

12 oz can of regular soda

3 chocolate sandwich cookies

Air-popped popcorn or dry-roasted nuts

8 oz sugar-free non-fat yogurt

Bottle of sparkling water

1 large orange

Beverage Swaps

16 ounce caffè latte w/whole milk

20-ounce bottle of regular cola

Vending machine sweetened iced tea (16 ounces)

A glass of regular ginger ale (12 ounces)

12 ounces caffè latte made with fat-free milk

Still or sparkling water

Water with a slice of lemon or lime

Sparkling water with a splash of 100% fruit juice

Beautifully
WELL

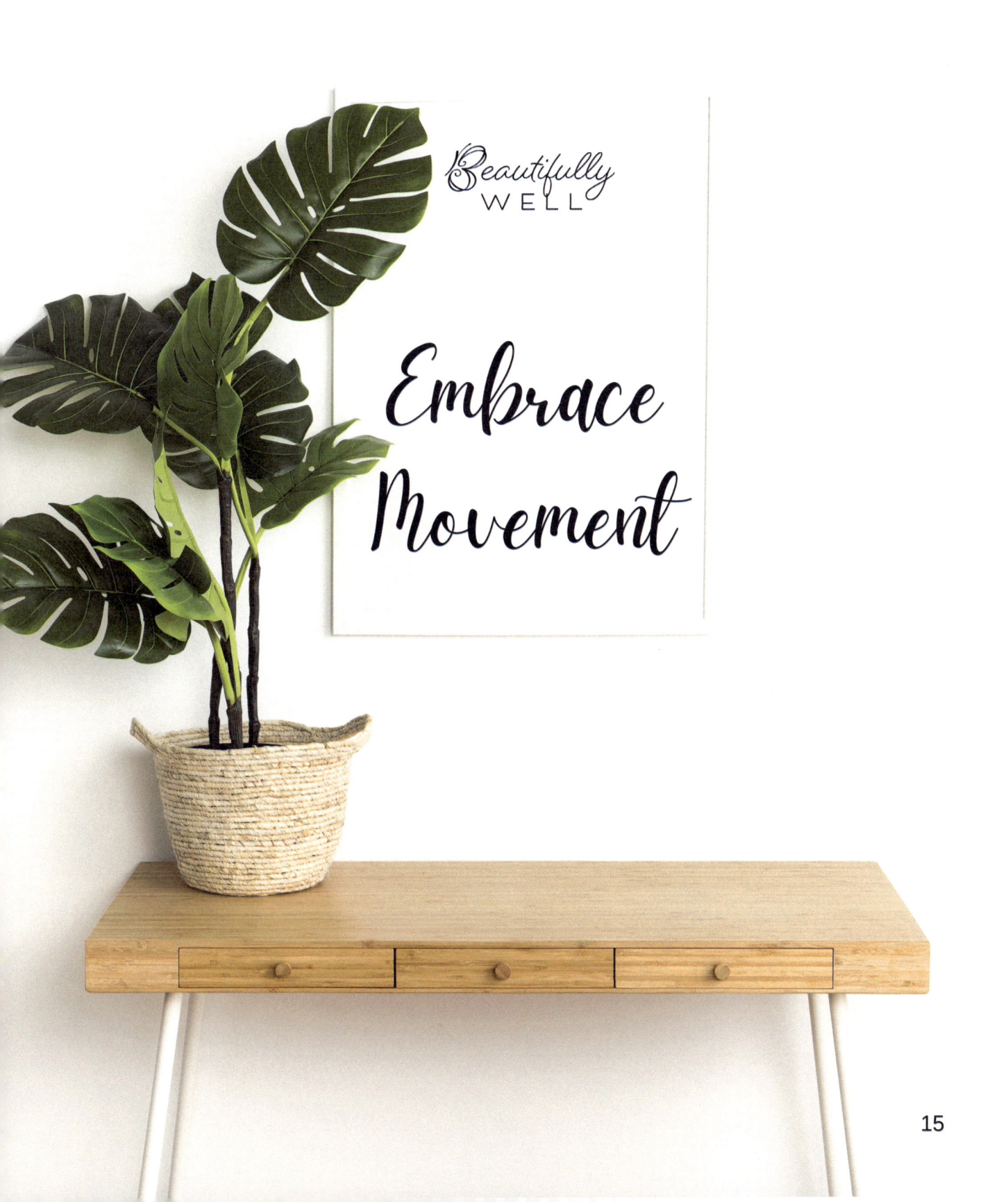

Embrace Movement

Angela's Rebound after a Setback....

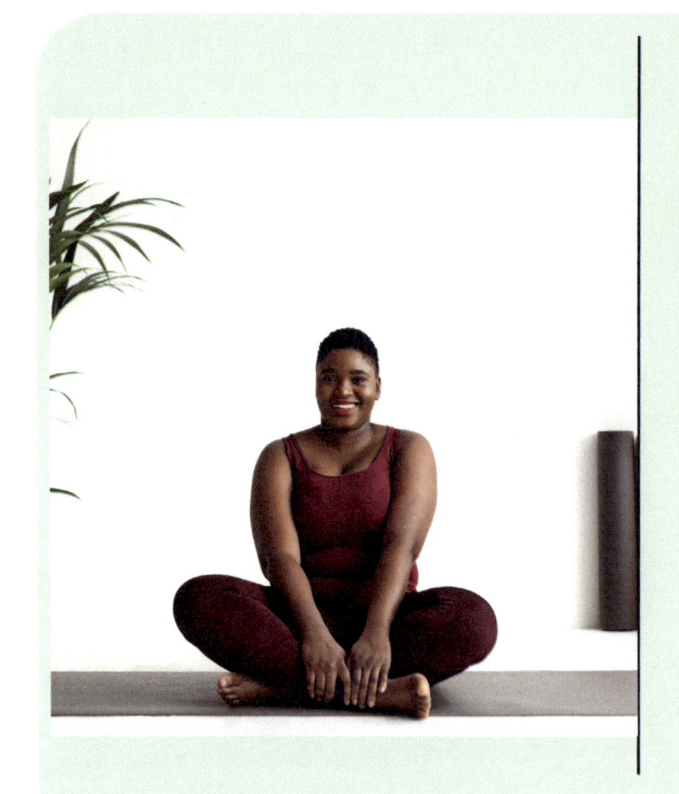

Angela just found out she has prediabetes. Her doctor asked her to lose 20 pounds and aim for at least 150 minutes of activity each week. She tries to meet this goal by walking for 30 minutes 5 days a week. With a lot of hard work, Angela reached her weight and activity goals. Her blood sugar levels are in the normal range now. And her doctor says she's lowered her risk for type 2 diabetes. Angela's doctor tells her to keep up the good work and reminds her of some of the benefits of staying active.

But as time goes on, Angela's schedule gets busier. Her husband starts going to night classes. So, in addition to preparing dinner on her scheduled days for the family, she needs to prepare dinner two additional days of the week. Angela now goes to the grocery store during her lunch break.

As a result, she no longer has time to walk during lunch. It's hard for Angela to find time to be active. Plus, she's met her weight loss goal, so she feels less motivated. Her physical activity routine is slipping. Angela decides to take action. She is active with her kids.

She gives herself small, non-food rewards for meeting her movement goals. And she asks her kids to pitch in more with preparing meals and other chores around the house, so she has more time to be active.

Today, Angela's physical activity routine is back on track. She plans to stay active over the long term. She wants to be healthy. Plus, she likes how she feels when she's active.

Ways to Get Active

There are so many ways to get active. Find at least one that you enjoy. Here are a few ideas.

1. After you read six pages of a book, get up and move a little.
2. Dance to your favorite music.
3. Pace the sidelines at your children's or grandchildren's sportse vents.
4. Play actively with your children or pets for 15 to 30 minutes a day.
5. Replace Sunday drives with Sunday walks.
6. Run or walk fast when you do errands.
7. Start a new active hobby, such as biking or hiking.
8. Take a walk after dinner with your family or by yourself.
9. Track your steps with a pedometer. Work up to 10,000 steps or more a day.
10. Walk around whenever you talk on the phone.
11. Walk briskly when you shop.
12. Walk up and down escalators instead of just riding them.
13. Walk your dog each day.
14. When you watch TV, stand up and move during the ads, or do chores.

Are You Ready to Get Active?

How do you plan to get active? Add your activity to your planning pages in this guide.

_____

_____

_____

_____

_____

_____

Be Active, Be Safe

Know what you can and cannot do based on your current health, then build up exercise activity from that point.

1. Ask your healthcare provider if you are ready to be active.
2. Dress in the right clothing for the activity. Use safety gear as needed.
3. Drink water before, during, and after your workout.
4. Slow down or stop if you feel very tired, sick, or faint, or your joints hurt.
5. Do a variety of activities to avoid straining anyone part of your body.
6. Start small. Try to make slow, steady progress over time.
7. Warm up before you work out. Cool down after you work out. Take 5 to 10 minutes for each.
8. Be careful not to trip or bump into anything.
9. Work out indoors if it's too hot or too cold. If you get too hot, you may experience headache, fast heartbeat, dizziness, stomach sickness, or feel faint.
10. Use good form when strength training.

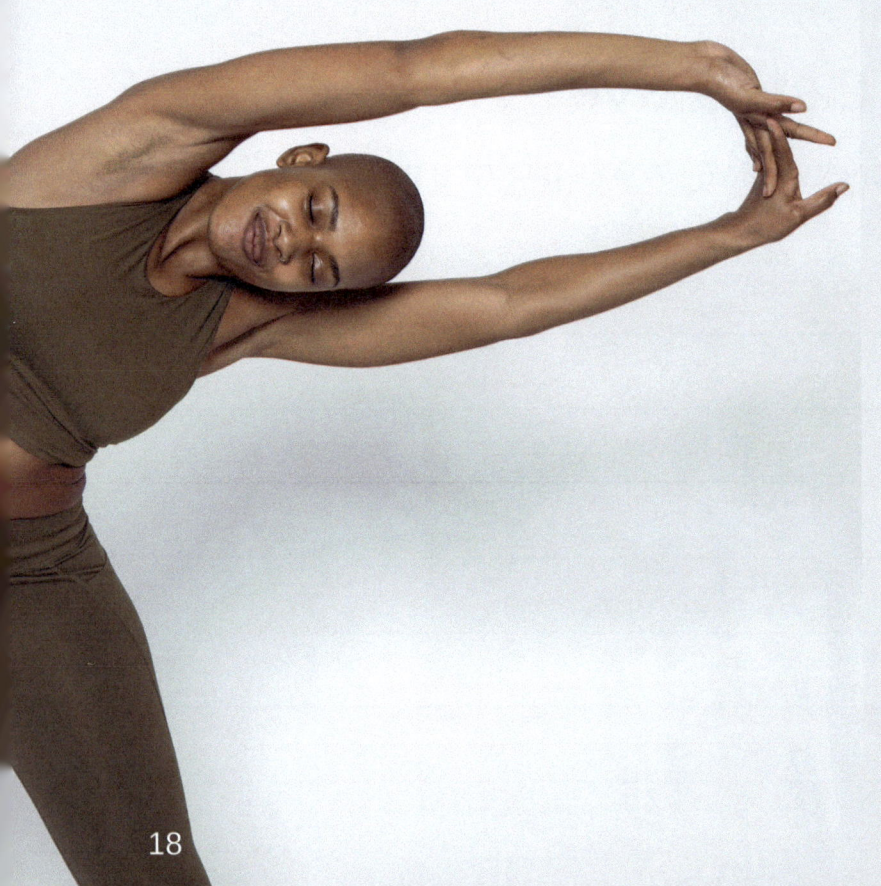

Source: National Institute of Aging/National Institutes of Health: Staying Safe During Exercise and Physical Activity (https:// go4life.nia.nih.gov/sites/default/files/Stay-ingSafe.pdf) Harvard Health Publications (http://www.health.harvard.edu/health-beat/10-tips-for-exercising-safely)

How many calories does activity burn?

This chart shows about how many calories a person who weighs 154 pounds would burn at a moderate pace.

Calories burned at a moderate pace

Activities	In 1 Hour	30 Minutes
Hiking	370	185
Light gardening/yard work	330	165
Dancing	330	165
Golf	330	165
Bicycling	290	145
Walking	280	140
Weight training (general light workout)	220	110
Stretching	180	90

Source: US Department of Agriculture. MyPlate.(http://www.choosemyplate.gov/physical-activity-calories-burn)

Weekly Plans

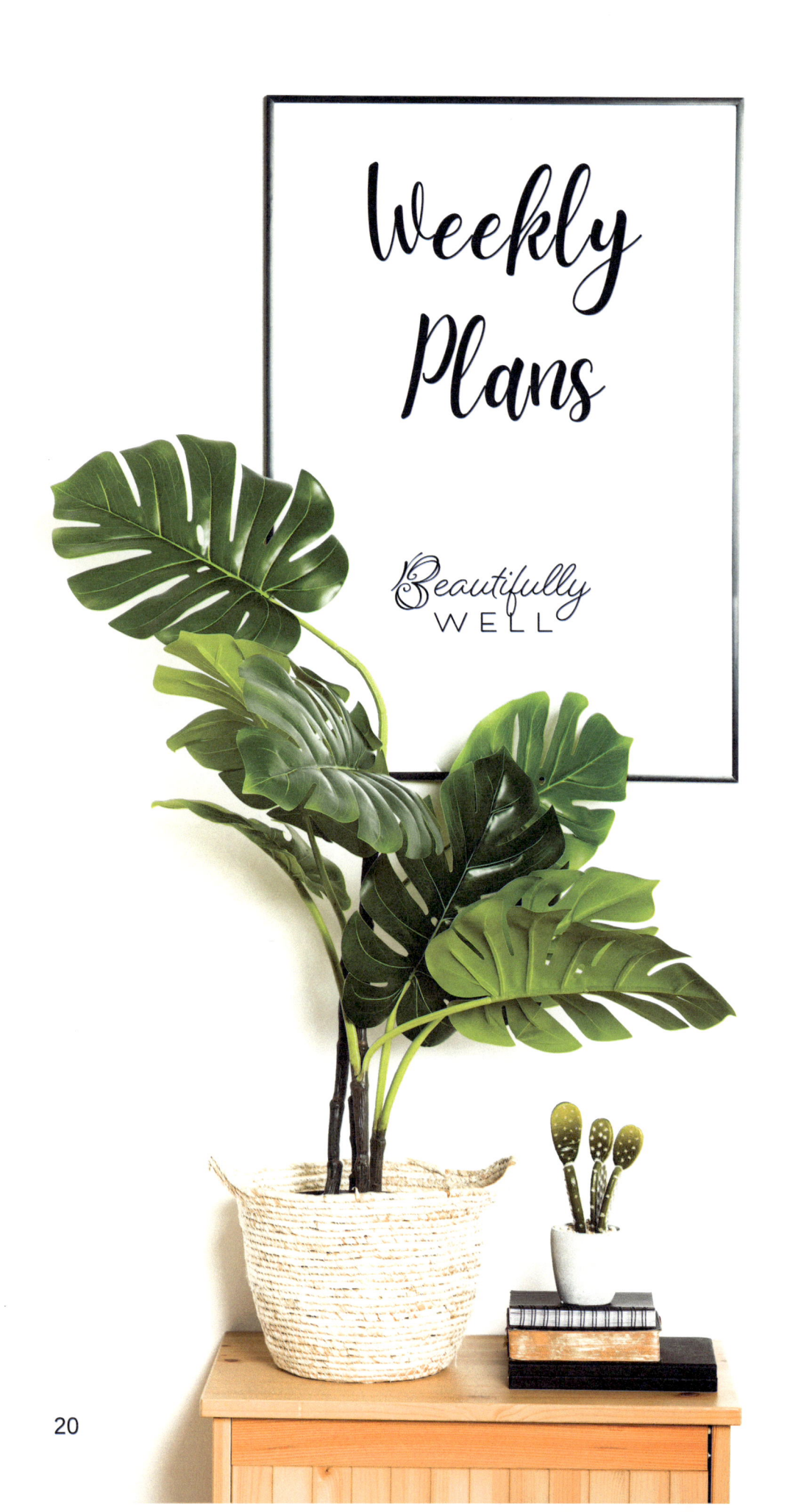

Beautifully WELL

Plan for Success

Set a goal to work on between now and the next session. The goal should help you improve your health. Write three actions you will take to reach it. Then check off each action you complete.

*Tips for Making Your Action Plan
Making an action plan can help you prevent type 2 diabetes.

REMEMBER:

1. Be realistic. Plan actions that are realistic for you.
2. Make it doable. Plan small changes. Over time, these changes will add up.
3. Be specific. Plan your actions in detail.

DECIDE:

What you will do

Where you will do it

When you will do it

How long you will do it

Be flexible. Review your action plan often. Look for ways to cope with challenges. If your action plan isn't working for you, revise it. Focus on behaviors. For instance, you can control how many pounds you lose by focusing on your actions, such as what you eat and how active you are. Make it enjoyable. Change doesn't have to be painful. Find activities and healthy foods that you enjoy.

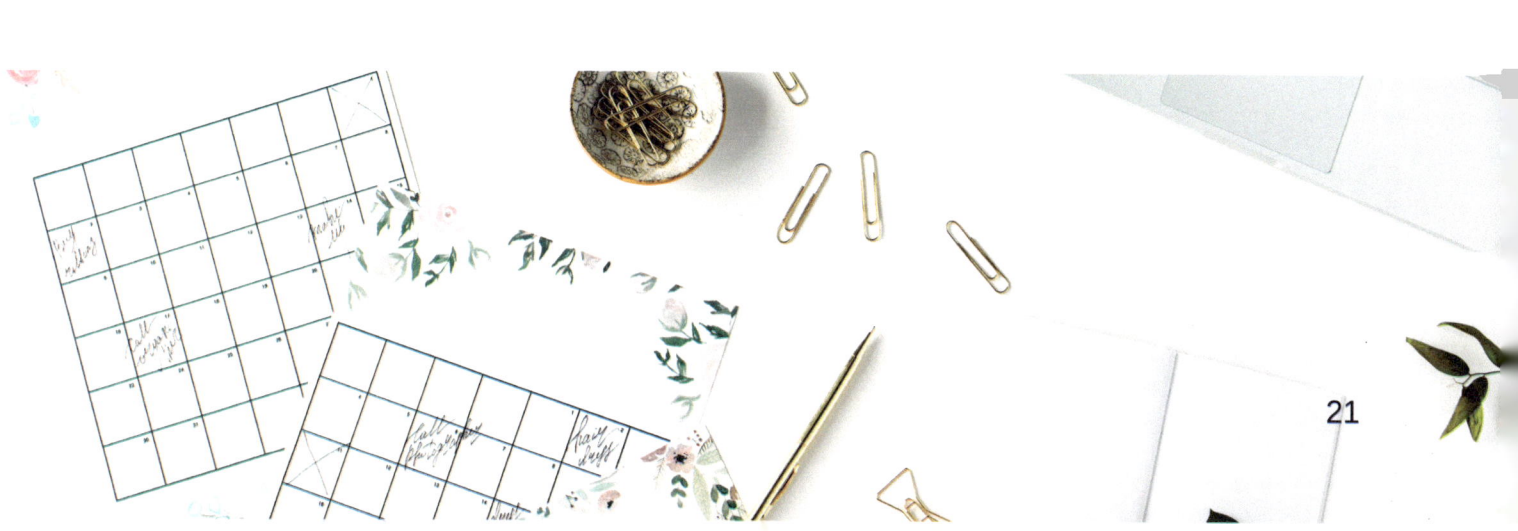

What I Envision This Month

Fitness

Food

Stress

WEEK 1

Current Weight: _____

My focus for this week:

_____

What I will do:

_____

Where and when will I do it:

_____

How long will I do it:

_____

Challenge I might face:

_____

Ways to cope with the challenge:

_____

_____

My non-food reward for accomplishing the goal:

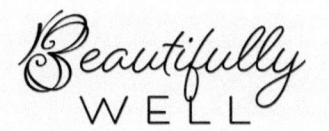

_____

_____

Let Today be the Start of Something New

WEEKLY PLANNER

FOR THE WEEK OF: _____

	BREAKFAST	LUNCH	DINNER	SNACKS	WATER
MON					💧💧💧💧
TUE					💧💧💧💧
WED					💧💧💧💧
THU					💧💧💧💧
FRI					💧💧💧💧
SAT					💧💧💧💧
SUN					💧💧💧💧

Shopping List:

_____

_____

_____

EXERCISE / ACTIVITY

WEEK 2

Current Weight: _____

My focus for this week:

_____

What I will do:

_____

Where and when will I do it:

_____

How long will I do it:

_____

Challenge I might face:

_____

Ways to cope with the challenge:

_____

_____

My non-food reward for accomplishing the goal:

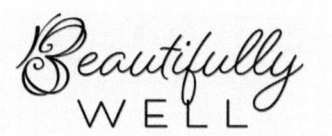

_____

_____

Beautifully WELL **Don't Dream of Success, Work for it!**

WEEKLY PLANNER

FOR THE WEEK OF: _____

	BREAKFAST	LUNCH	DINNER	SNACKS	WATER
MON					💧💧💧💧
TUE					💧💧💧💧
WED					💧💧💧💧
THU					💧💧💧💧
FRI					💧💧💧💧
SAT					💧💧💧💧
SUN					💧💧💧💧

Shopping List:

_____

_____

_____

EXERCISE / ACTIVITY

WEEK 3

Current Weight: _____

My focus for this week:

_____

What I will do:

_____

Where and when will I do it:

_____

How long will I do it:

_____

Challenge I might face:

_____

Ways to cope with the challenge:

_____
_____

My non-food reward for accomplishing the goal:

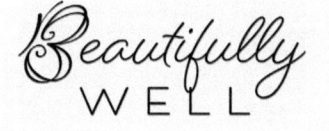

_____
_____

Beautifully WELL   **H.O.P.E. Have Only Positive Expectations.**

WEEKLY PLANNER

FOR THE WEEK OF: _____

	BREAKFAST	LUNCH	DINNER	SNACKS	WATER
MON					◊◊◊◊
TUE					◊◊◊◊
WED					◊◊◊◊
THU					◊◊◊◊
FRI					◊◊◊◊
SAT					◊◊◊◊
SUN					◊◊◊◊

Shopping List:

_____

_____

_____

EXERCISE / ACTIVITY

WEEK 4

Current Weight: _____

My focus for this week:

_____

What I will do:

_____

Where and when will I do it:

_____

How long will I do it:

_____

Challenge I might face:

_____

Ways to cope with the challenge:

_____

_____

My non-food reward for accomplishing the goal:

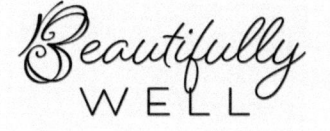

_____

_____

Progress is a Process

WEEKLY PLANNER

FOR THE WEEK OF: _____

	BREAKFAST	LUNCH	DINNER	SNACKS	WATER
MON					◊◊◊◊
TUE					◊◊◊◊
WED					◊◊◊◊
THU					◊◊◊◊
FRI					◊◊◊◊
SAT					◊◊◊◊
SUN					◊◊◊◊

Shopping List:

_____

_____

_____

EXERCISE / ACTIVITY

What I Accomplished This Month

Fitness

Food

Stress

Next Month's Goals

Fitness

Food

Stress

Bonus: Meal Planning

MEAL PLAN　　　　　　AMANI NICOL WELLNESS

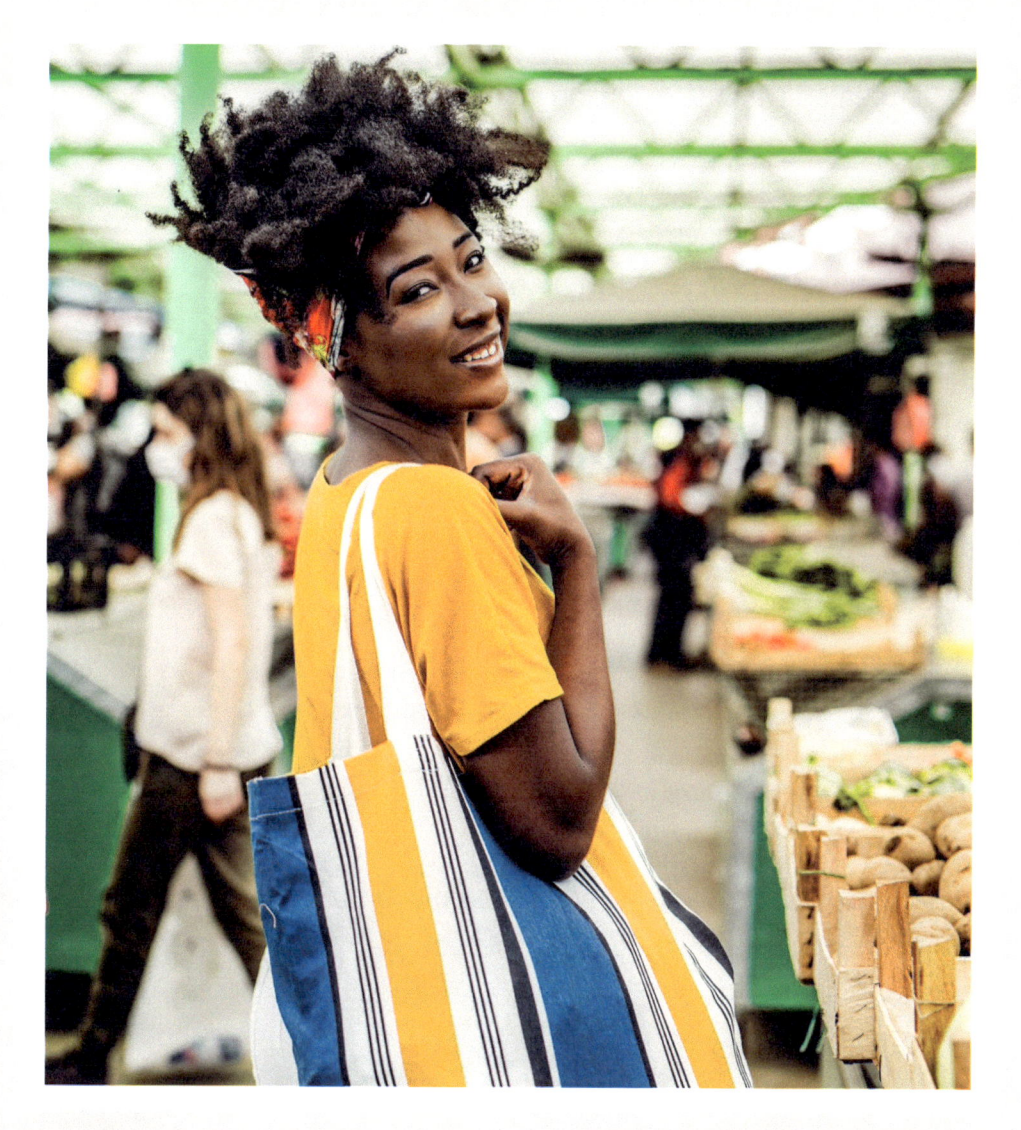

Weight Management

SIMPLY BALANCED

Simple Balanced Diet

This program helps teach balanced diet basics with a variety of delicious meals and easy-to-follow recipes. The plan is rich in whole grains, fruits, vegetables, lean proteins, and healthy fats. It limits sodium and added sugars. The meals included in this program support bone health and the immune system while also providing adequate iron intake.

This program was created with the following key considerations:

Macronutrients

An ideal diet meets food group needs with nutrient-dense options and comprises over 40% carbohydrates, 10% to 30% protein, and under 40% fat. This plan contains a variety of foods to provide adequate nutrition and fuel throughout the day.

Bone Building Nutrients

This meal plan uses calcium- rich ingredients like fortified milk beverages, Greek yogurt, and chia seeds. Magnesium is incorporated from food sources like chickpeas and leafy greens.

Iron

Iron is an important mineral that helps produce red blood cells and transport oxygen throughout the body. This meal plan provides iron sources like poultry, ground beef, and spinach.

Immune Support

The plan provides over 80 mcg of selenium daily by incorporating eggs, beef, oats, and bananas. The plan includes vitamin C from whole food sources like strawberries, broccoli, and bell pepper.

Christi Dorsey

Registered Dietician
CEO of Taste Symmetry

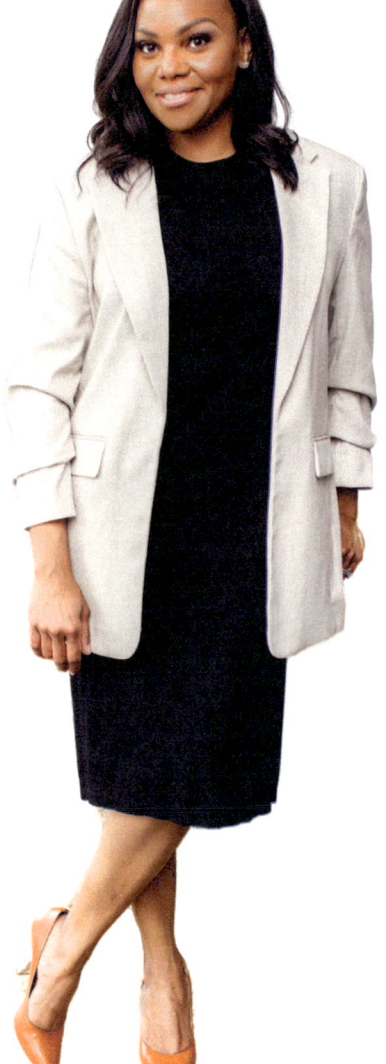

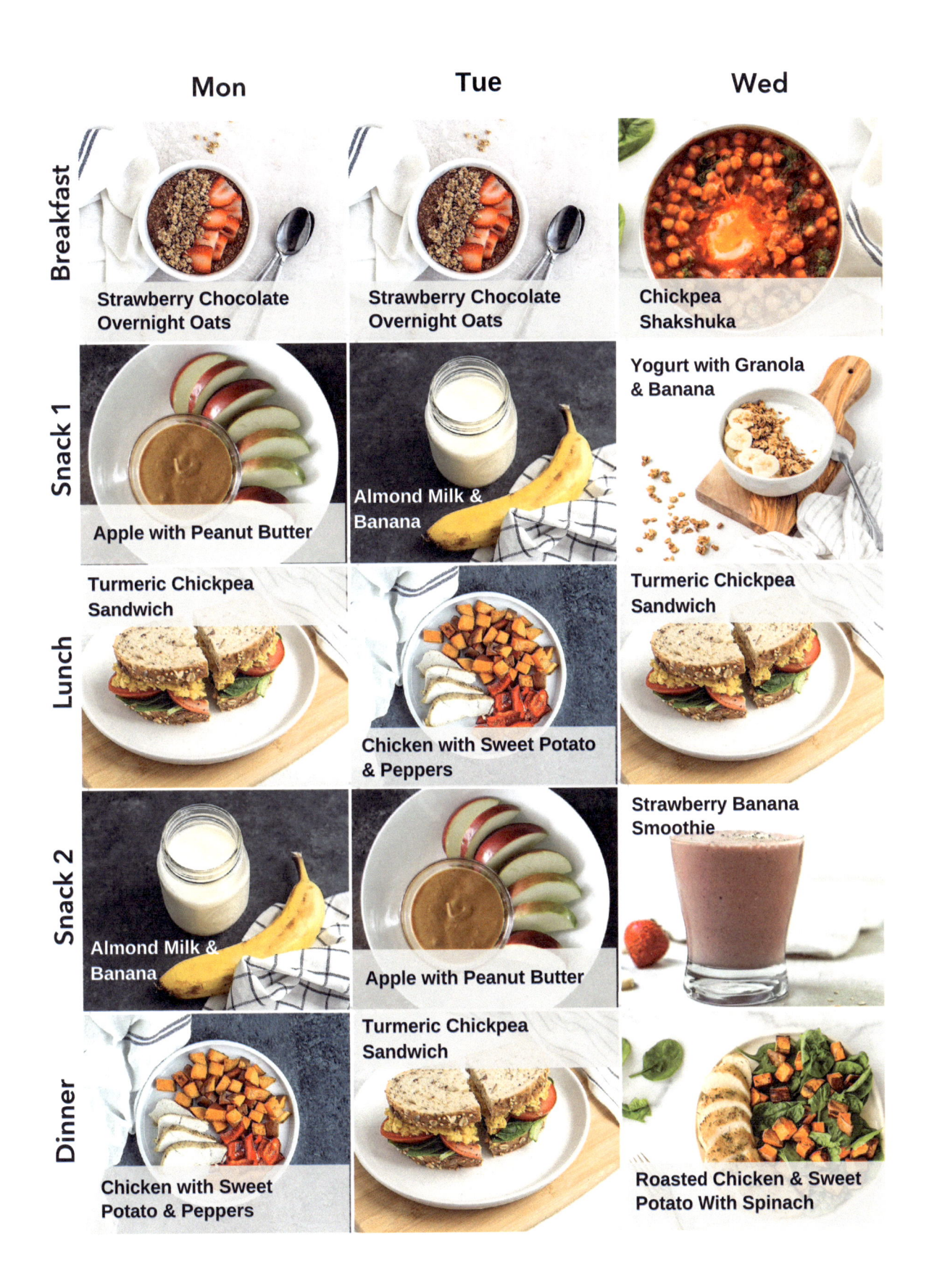

	Mon	Tue	Wed
Breakfast	Strawberry Chocolate Overnight Oats	Strawberry Chocolate Overnight Oats	Chickpea Shakshuka
Snack 1	Apple with Peanut Butter	Almond Milk & Banana	Yogurt with Granola & Banana
Lunch	Turmeric Chickpea Sandwich	Chicken with Sweet Potato & Peppers	Turmeric Chickpea Sandwich
Snack 2	Almond Milk & Banana	Apple with Peanut Butter	Strawberry Banana Smoothie
Dinner	Chicken with Sweet Potato & Peppers	Turmeric Chickpea Sandwich	Roasted Chicken & Sweet Potato With Spinach

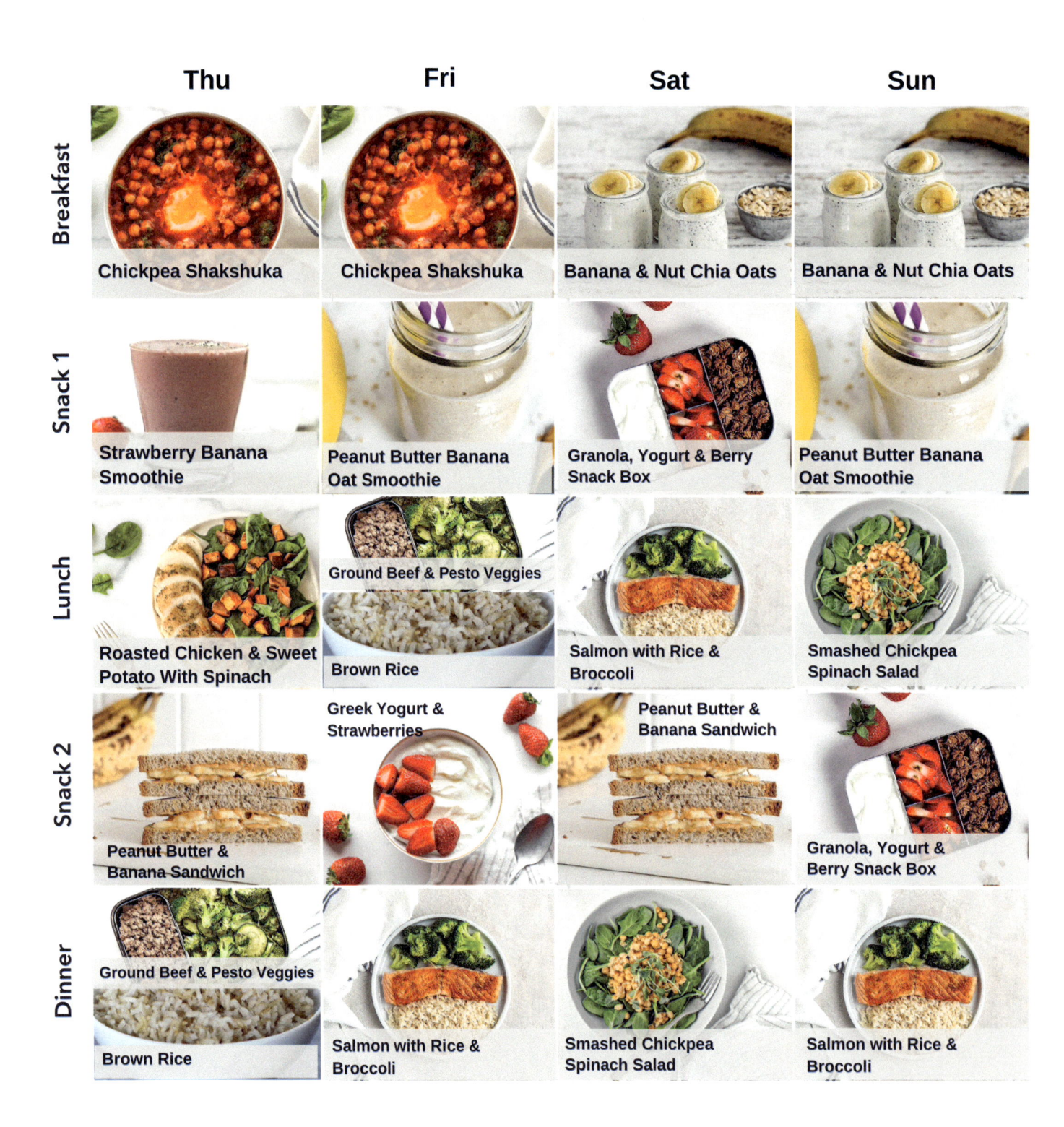

	Thu	Fri	Sat	Sun
Breakfast	Chickpea Shakshuka	Chickpea Shakshuka	Banana & Nut Chia Oats	Banana & Nut Chia Oats
Snack 1	Strawberry Banana Smoothie	Peanut Butter Banana Oat Smoothie	Granola, Yogurt & Berry Snack Box	Peanut Butter Banana Oat Smoothie
Lunch	Roasted Chicken & Sweet Potato With Spinach	Ground Beef & Pesto Veggies / Brown Rice	Salmon with Rice & Broccoli	Smashed Chickpea Spinach Salad
Snack 2	Peanut Butter & Banana Sandwich	Greek Yogurt & Strawberries	Peanut Butter & Banana Sandwich	Granola, Yogurt & Berry Snack Box
Dinner	Ground Beef & Pesto Veggies / Brown Rice	Salmon with Rice & Broccoli	Smashed Chickpea Spinach Salad	Salmon with Rice & Broccoli

Shopping List

Fruits

- 2 Apple
- 8 Banana
- 1 Lemon
- 5 1/2 cups Strawberries

Breakfast

- 3/4 cup All Natural Peanut Butter
- 1 1/2 cups Granola
- 2 2/3 tbsps Maple Syrup

Seeds, Nuts & Spices

- 2 tbsps Chia Seeds
- 1 tsp Garlic Powder
- 1 tbsp Harissa
- 2 tbsps Hemp Seeds
- 1/2 tsp Paprika
- 0 Sea Salt & Black Pepper
- 1/2 tsp Turmeric

Shopping List

Vegetables

- [ ] **10 cups** Baby Spinach
- [ ] **5 cups** Broccoli
- [ ] **1** Garlic
- [ ] **1/2 cup** Microgreens
- [ ] **1** Red Bell Pepper
- [ ] **2** Sweet Potato
- [ ] **1 tsp** Thyme
- [ ] **1** Tomato
- [ ] **1** Zucchini

Boxed & Canned

- [ ] **1 1/4 cups** Brown Rice
- [ ] **6 1/2 cups** Chickpeas
- [ ] **3/4 cup** Tomato Purée

Baking

- [ ] **2 tbsps** Cocoa Powder
- [ ] **2 cups** Oats
- [ ] **1 tsp** Vanilla Extract

Shopping List

Bread, Fish, Meat & Cheese

- 1 1/4 lbs   Chicken Breast
- 8 ozs   Lean Ground Beef
- 1 1/8 lbs   Salmon Fillet
- 10 slices   Whole Grain Bread

Condiments & Oils

- 3 3/4 tbsps   Extra Virgin Olive Oil
- 1 tbsp   Pesto
- 1/3 cup   Vegan Mayonnaise

Cold

- 3   Eggs
- 3 1/2 cups   Plain Greek Yogurt
- 7 cups   Unsweetened Almond Milk

Other

- 1 cup   Water

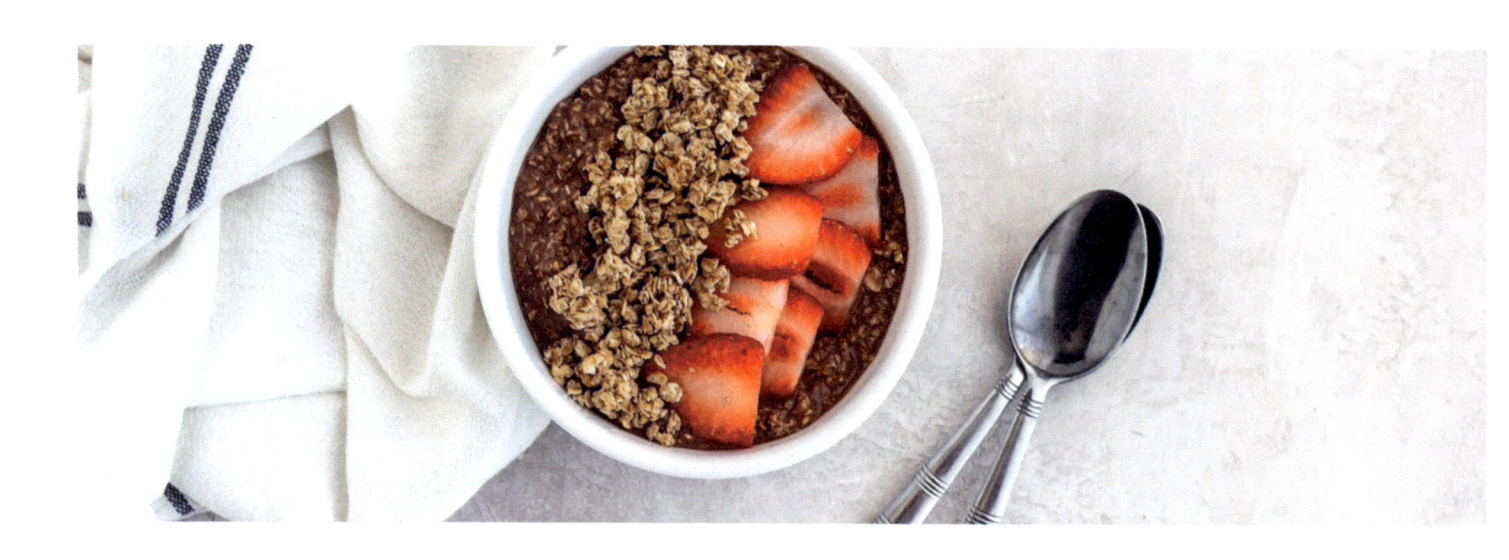

Strawberry Chocolate Overnight Oats

2 servings
3 hours 5 minutes

Ingredients

1 cup   Oats (quick or rolled)
1 cup   Unsweetened Almond Milk
2 tbsps   Maple Syrup
2 tbsps   Cocoa Powder
1 cup   Strawberries (sliced or chopped)
1/2 cup   Granola (optional)

Directions

1. Combine the oats, milk, maple syrup, and cocoa powder in a bowl. Stir well. Cover and refrigerate for at least three hours or overnight.

2. To serve, divide the oats between bowls or jars and top with the strawberries and granola (if using). Enjoy!

Notes

Leftovers: Refrigerate in an airtight container for up to three days. Top with strawberries and granola just before serving.

Serving Size: One serving is approximately equal to 3/4 cup of the oats.

Nut-Free: Use a nut-free milk, like coconut milk or cow's milk.

More Flavor: Add cinnamon, vanilla, or a pinch of salt.

No Strawberries: Use another berry or banana slices instead.

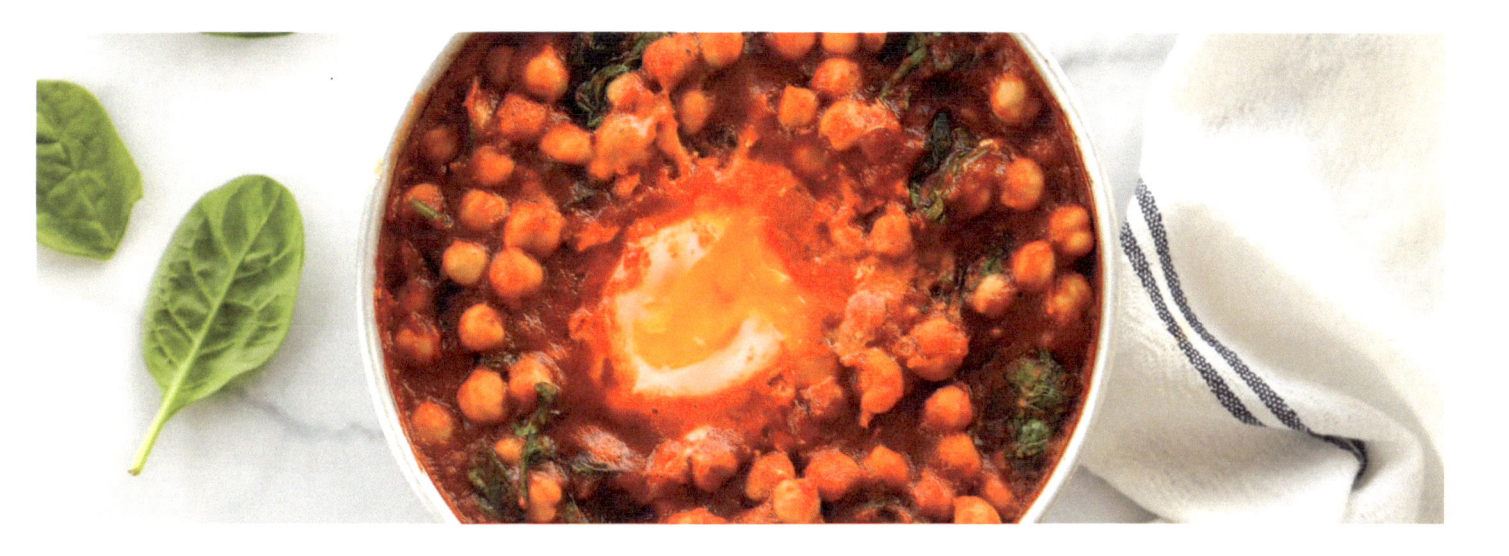

Chickpea Shakshuka

3 servings
15 minutes

Ingredients

3 cups Chickpeas (cooked)
3/4 cup Tomato Purée
1 tbsp Harissa
1 1/2 cups Baby Spinach
3 Eggs
Sea Salt & Black Pepper (to taste)

Directions

1. In a small pan over medium heat add the chickpeas, tomato purée, and harissa. Bring to boil, reduce the heat down to simmer, and let cook for about 10 minutes.

2. Add the spinach and cook for another two minutes. Create a pocket in the middle and crack the egg into the pocket. Cover the pan and cook until the egg is set, about five to six minutes.

3. Season with salt and pepper and enjoy!

Notes

Leftovers: Refrigerate in an airtight container for up to three days.
Serving Size: One serving is equal to approximately 1 1/2 cups.
More Flavor: Add onion and bell pepper.
Additional Toppings: Add feta cheese and fresh herbs.

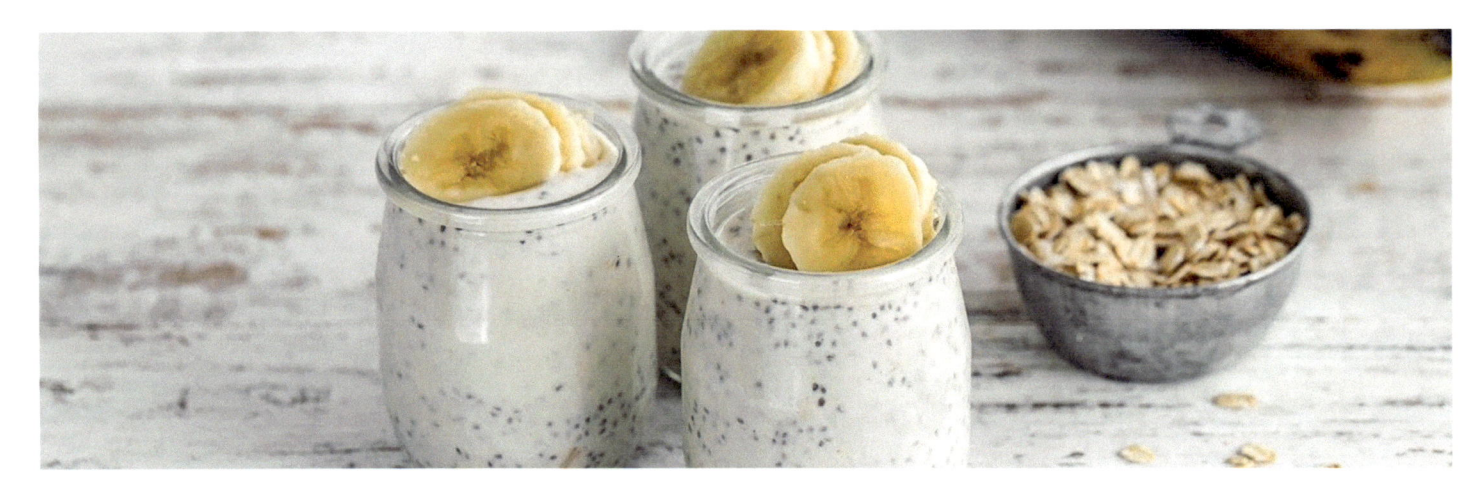

Banana & Nut Chia Oats

2 servings
8 hours

Ingredients

- 1 cup   Plain Greek Yogurt
- 1 cup   Unsweetened Almond Milk
- 2 tbsps   Oats (rolled)
- 2 tbsps   Chia Seeds
- 2 tsps   All Natural Peanut Butter
- 2 tsps   Maple Syrup
- 1 tsp   Vanilla Extract
- 1   Banana (sliced)

Directions

1. In a medium bowl, mix together the yogurt, almond milk, oats, chia seeds, peanut butter, maple syrup, and vanilla. Seal and place in the fridge overnight, or for at least eight hours.

2. Divide into containers and add the sliced banana. Serve and enjoy!

Notes

Leftovers: Refrigerate in a sealed container for up to four days.

Nut-Free: Use a nut-free milk such as oat or soy.

More Flavor: Add a pinch of cinnamon.

No Banana: Use mixed berries instead of banana.

Make it Vegan: Use a vegan yogurt.

Consistency: For a thicker consistency, add more chia seeds.

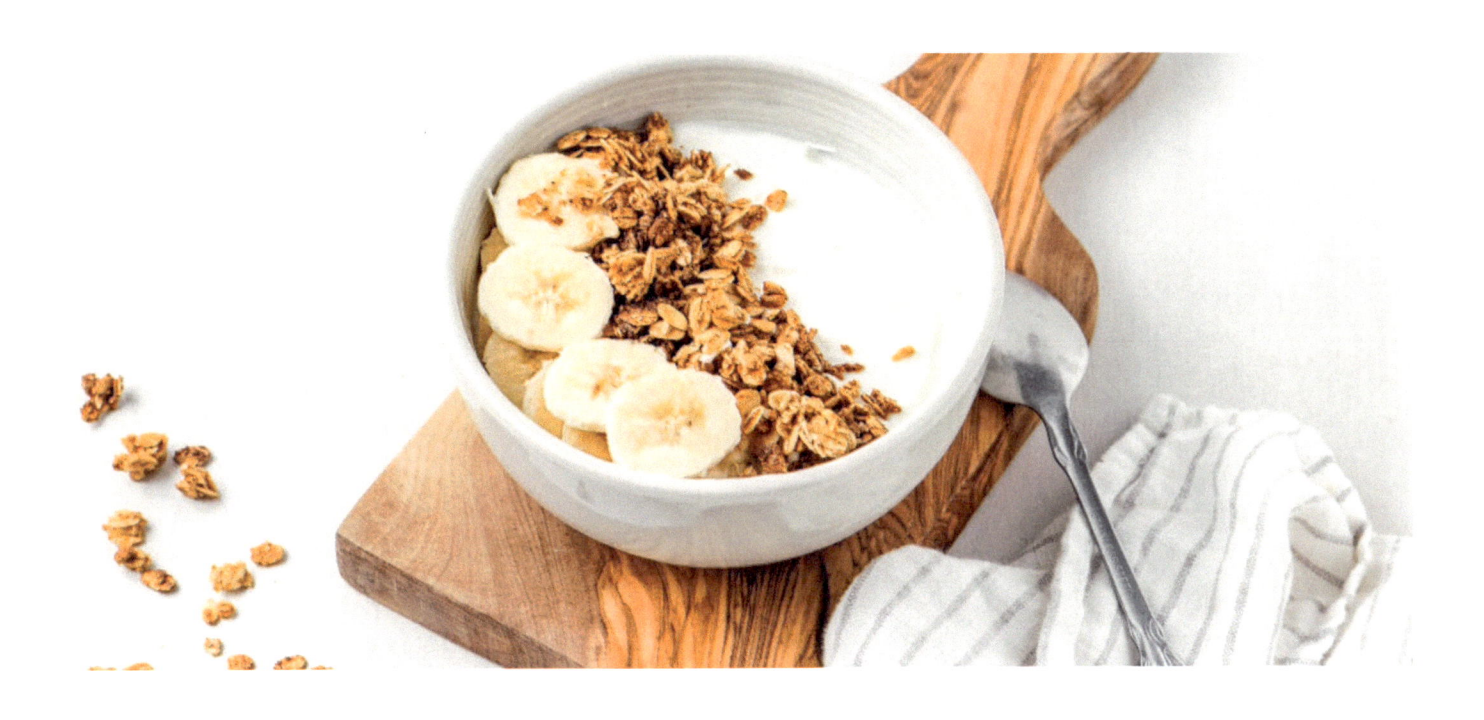

Yogurt with Granola & Banana

1 serving
5 minutes

Ingredients

1 cup Plain Greek Yogurt

1 Banana (sliced)

1/3 cup Granola

Directions

1. Add the yogurt, banana, and granola to a bowl, and enjoy!

Notes

More Flavor: Add maple syrup or vanilla.

Additional Toppings: Nut butter, shredded coconut, chia seeds, and/or hemp seeds.

Gluten-Free: Use gluten-free granola.

Dairy-Free: Use a dairy-free yogurt alternative.

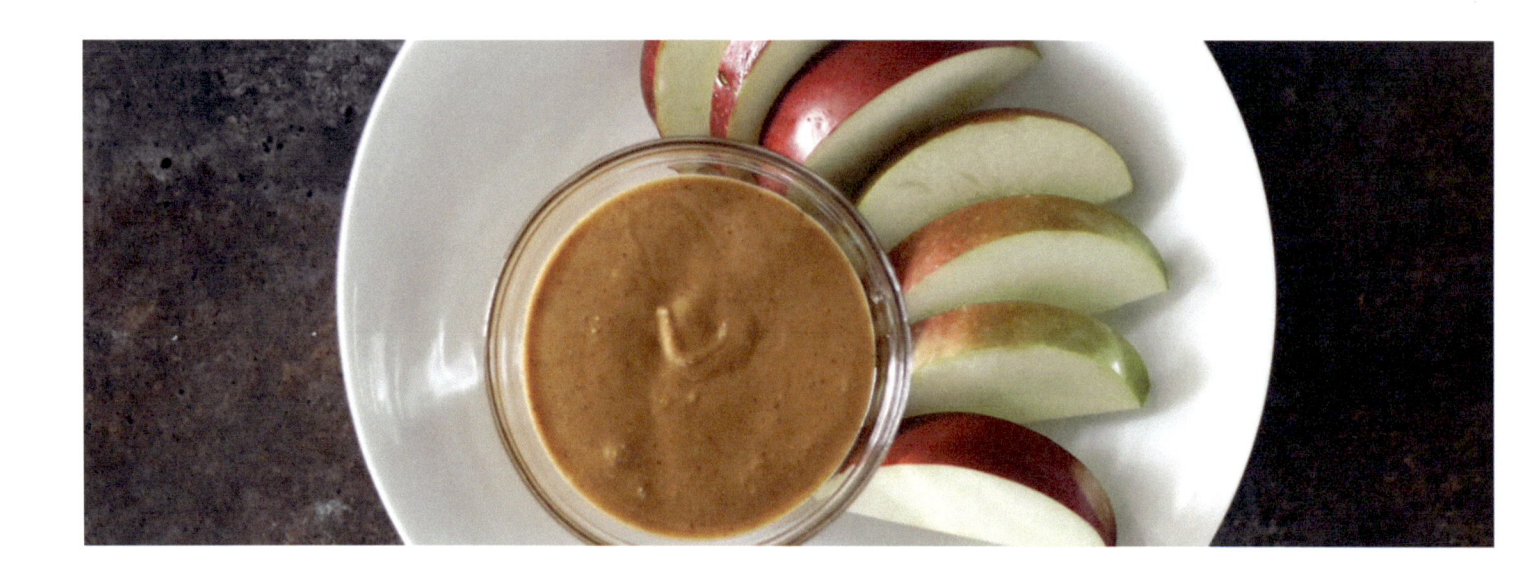

Apple with Peanut Butter

1 serving
3 minutes

Ingredients

1 Apple

2 tbsps All Natural Peanut Butter

Directions

1 Cut apple into slices and remove the core. Dip into peanut butter and enjoy!

Notes

Keep it Fresh: To avoid brown apple slices, assemble the slices back into the shape of the apple and tie an elastic band around it.

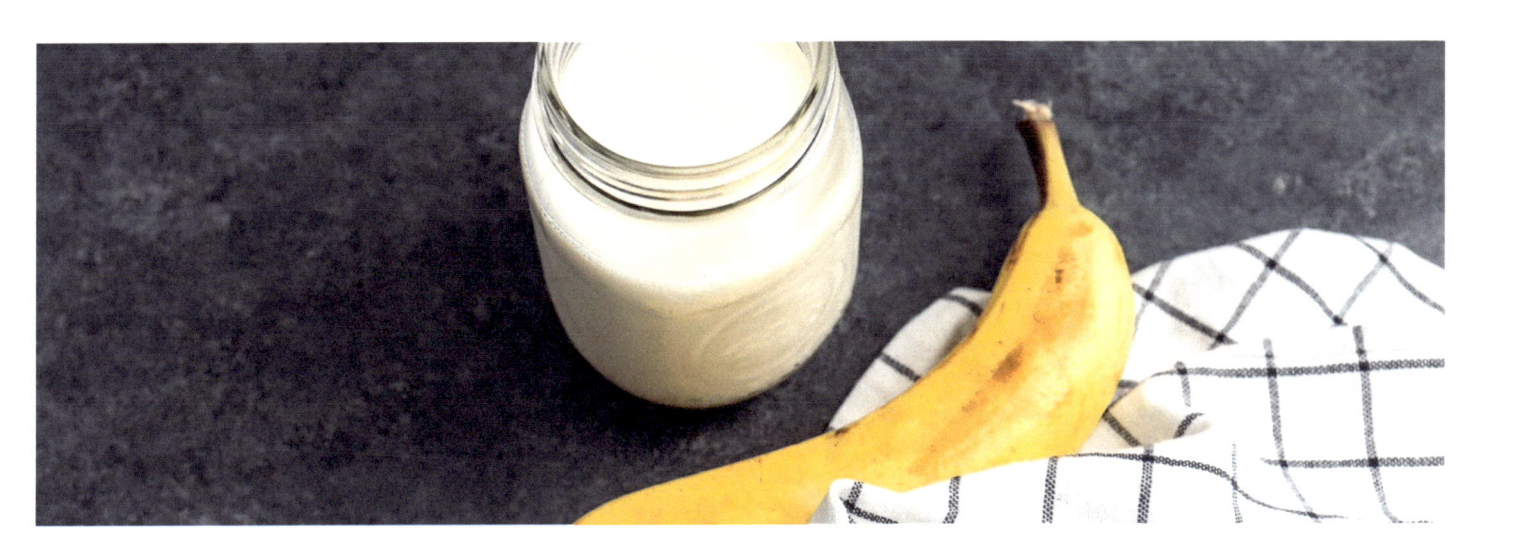

Almond Milk & Banana

1 serving
5 minutes

Ingredients

1 cup Unsweetened Almond Milk

1 Banana

Directions

1. Serve the almond milk with the banana. Enjoy!

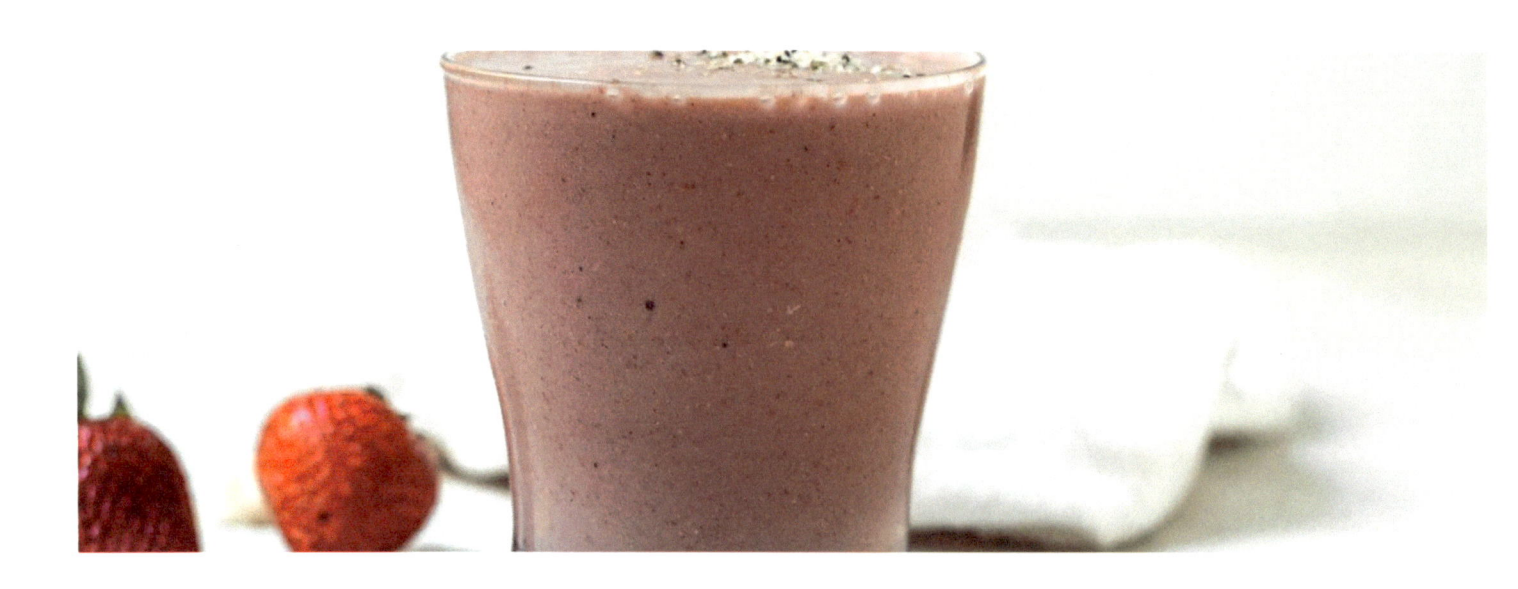

Strawberry Banana Smoothie

1 serving
5 minutes

Ingredients

1 cup Strawberries

1/2 Banana

2 tbsps Oats (quick or rolled)

1 cup Unsweetened Almond Milk

1 tbsp Hemp Seeds

Directions

1. Place all ingredients in your blender and blend until smooth. Pour into a glass and enjoy!

Notes

No Banana: Sweeten with raw honey, maple syrup or soaked dates instead.

Storage: Refrigerate in a sealed mason jar up to 48 hours.

More Protein: Add more hemp seeds, a scoop of protein powder, or a spoonful of nut butter.

More Fibre: Add ground flax seeds.

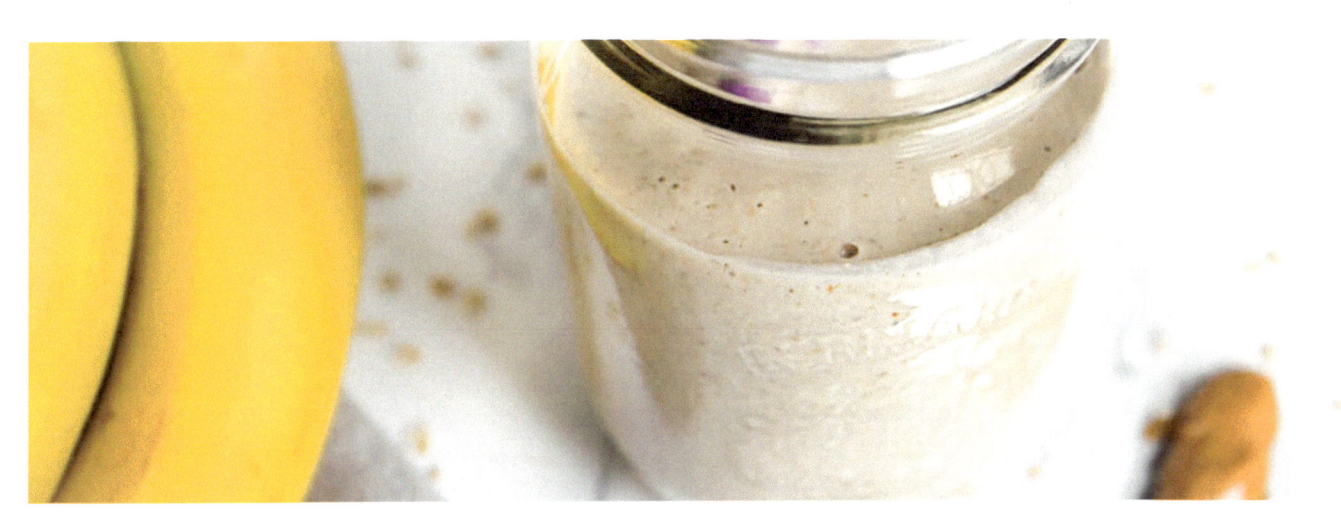

Peanut Butter Banana Oat Smoothie

1 serving
5 minutes

Ingredients

- 1/4 cup Oats (quick or traditional)
- 2 tbsps All Natural Peanut Butter
- 1 Banana
- 1/2 cup Unsweetened Almond Milk

Directions

1. Place all ingredients into a blender and blend well until smooth. Divide into glasses and enjoy! (Note: This smoothie will thicken if not had right away. Just add a splash of almond milk until you reach your desired consistency.)

Notes

No Banana: Sweeten with raw honey, maple syrup or a few soaked dates.

No Peanut Butter: Use any nut or seed butter.

Storage: Store in a mason jar with lid in the fridge up to 48 hours.

More Protein: Add hemp seeds or a scoop of protein powder.

More Fibre: Add ground flax seed.

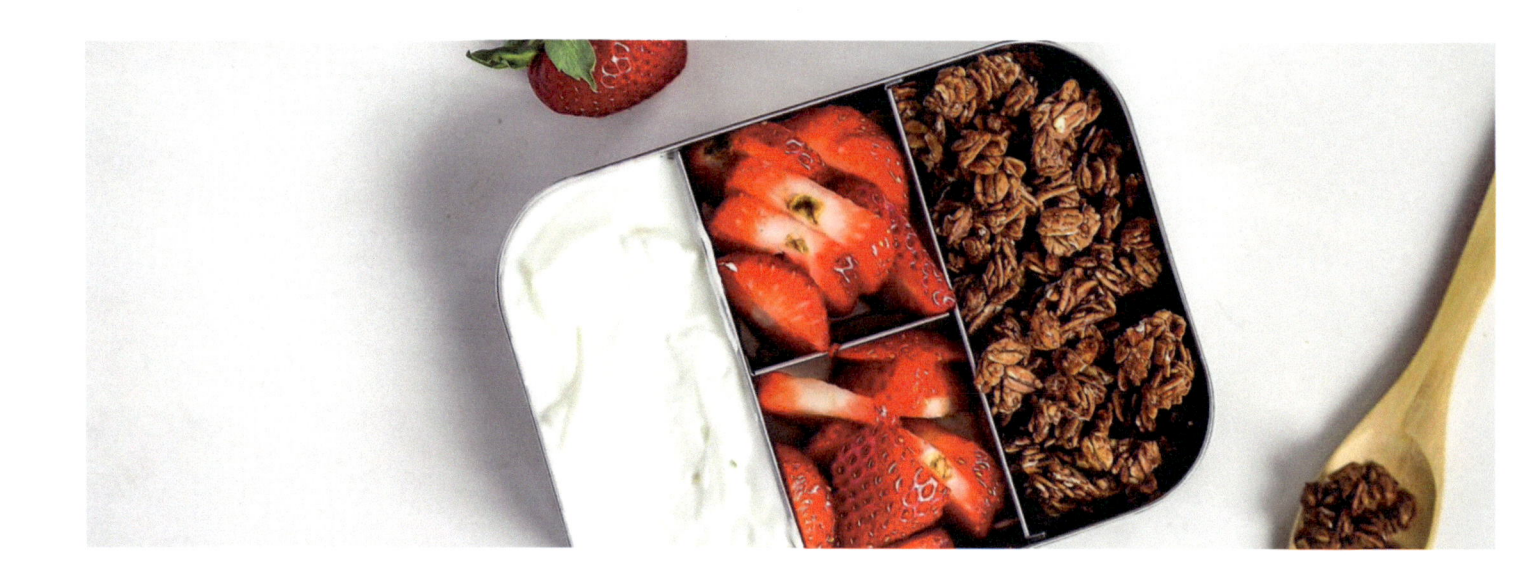

Granola, Yogurt & Berry Snack Box

1 serving
5 minutes

Ingredients

1/2 cup Plain Greek Yogurt
1 cup Strawberries (sliced)
1/3 cup Granola

Directions

1. Assemble all ingredients into a storage container and refrigerate until ready to eat. Enjoy!

Notes

Storage: Refrigerate in an airtight container up to 3 days.

Gluten-Free: Ensure a gluten-free granola is used.

Dairy-Free & Vegan: Use a dairy-free yogurt.

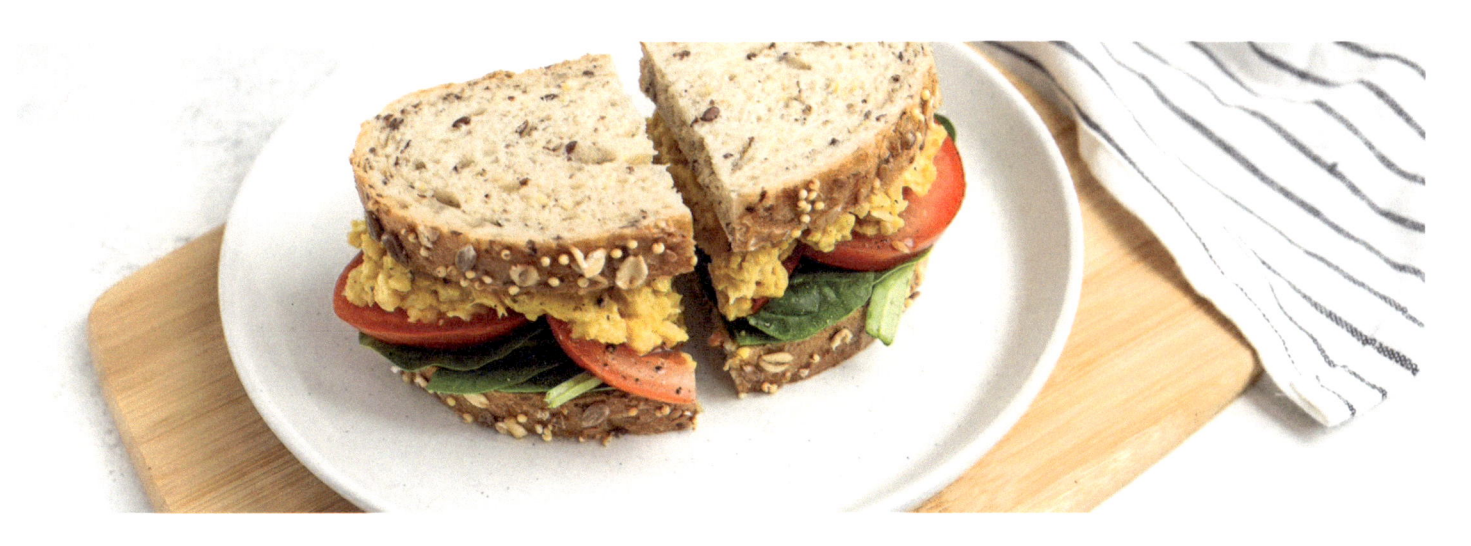

Turmeric Chickpea Sandwich

1 serving
10 minutes

Ingredients

2/3 cup	Chickpeas (cooked)
2 tbsps	Vegan Mayonnaise
1/8 tsp	Turmeric
2 slices	Whole Grain Bread
1/2 cup	Baby Spinach
1/3	Tomato (medium, sliced)

Sea Salt & Black Pepper (to taste)

Directions

1. Use the back of a fork to smash the chickpeas. Stir in the mayonnaise, turmeric, salt and pepper until well combined.

2. Scoop the turmeric chickpea mixture onto the bread. Add the spinach and tomato. Close the sandwich and enjoy!

Notes

Leftovers: Refrigerate in an airtight container for up to one day.

Gluten-Free: Use gluten-free bread instead.

More Flavor: Add onion powder and minced garlic. Toast the bread.

Additional Toppings: Add cucumber, sliced green onions, diced celery, or red onion.

Save Time: Blend the chickpeas, mayonnaise, turmeric, salt and pepper in a food processor to your desired consistency.

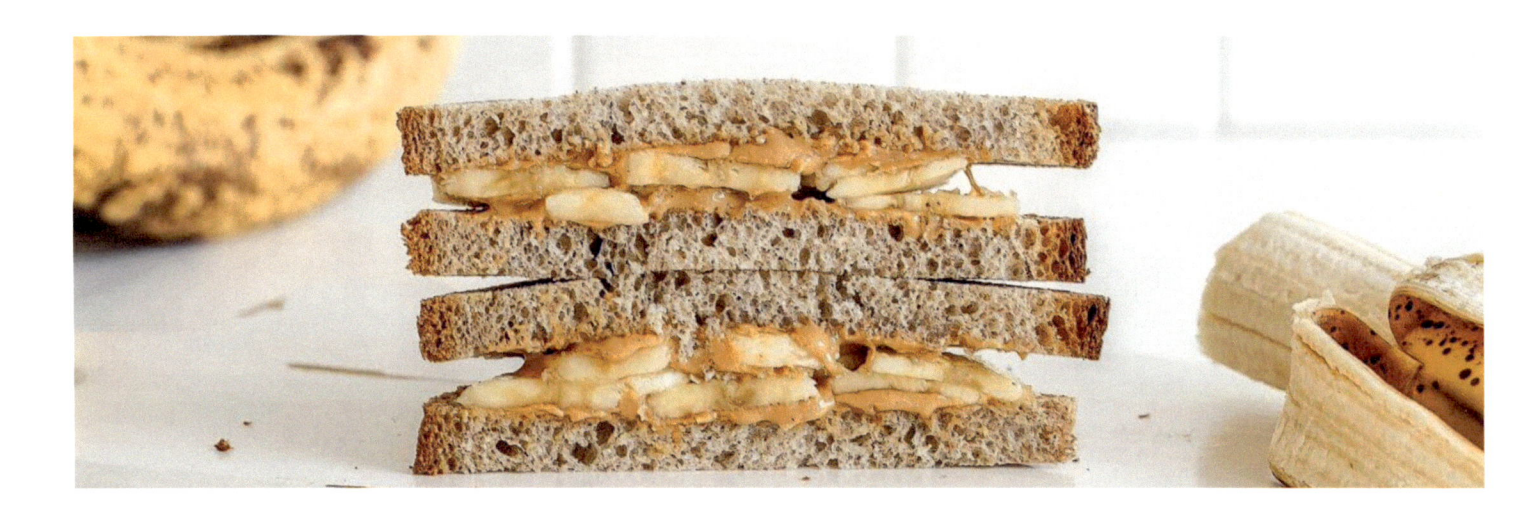

Peanut Butter & Banana Sandwich

1 serving
5 minutes

Ingredients

- **2 tbsps** All Natural Peanut Butter
- **2 slices** Whole Grain Bread
- **1/2** Banana (sliced into rounds)

Directions

1. Spread the peanut butter onto the bread. Top with bananas. Close the sandwich and slice. Enjoy!

Notes

Leftovers: Refrigerate in an airtight container for up to one day. Best enjoyed fresh.
More Flavor: Add a dash of cinnamon or drizzle of honey.
Gluten-Free: Use gluten-free bread.
Nut-Free: Use sunflower seed butter.

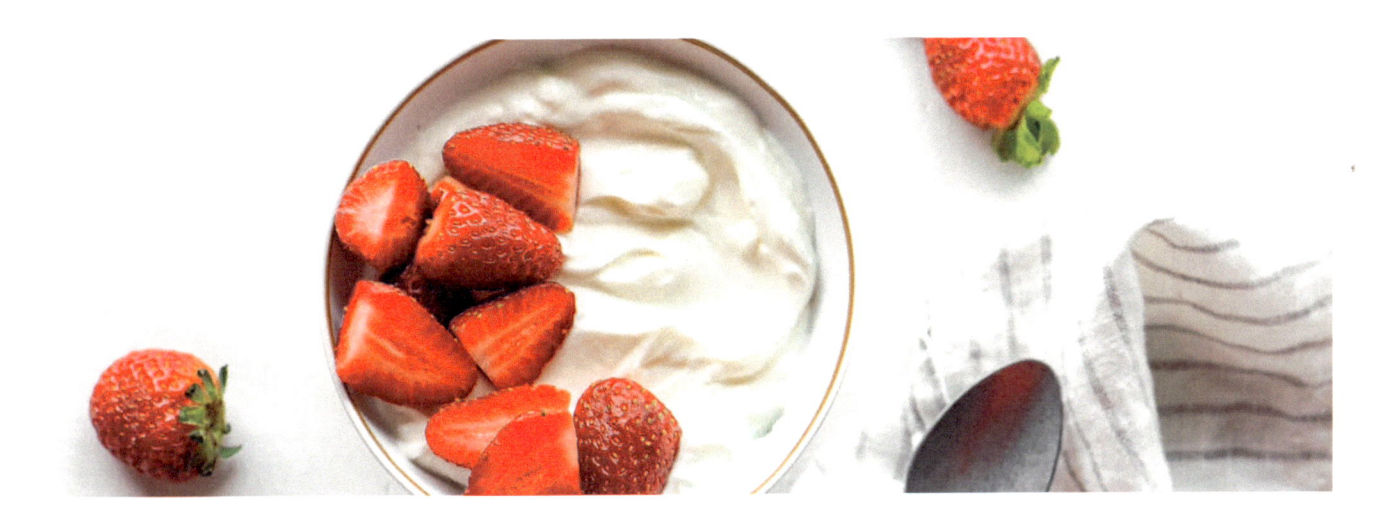

Greek Yogurt & Strawberries

1 serving
5 minutes

Ingredients

1/2 cup	Plain Greek Yogurt
1/2 cup	Strawberries

Directions

1 Add the yogurt to a bowl and top with strawberries. Enjoy!

Notes

Leftovers: Best enjoyed immediately or you can meal prep by storing in an airtight container for up to three days.

Make it Vegan: Use coconut yogurt instead of Greek yogurt.

More Flavor: Add maple syrup or honey.

Additional Toppings: Top with coconut flakes, granola, nuts, and seeds.

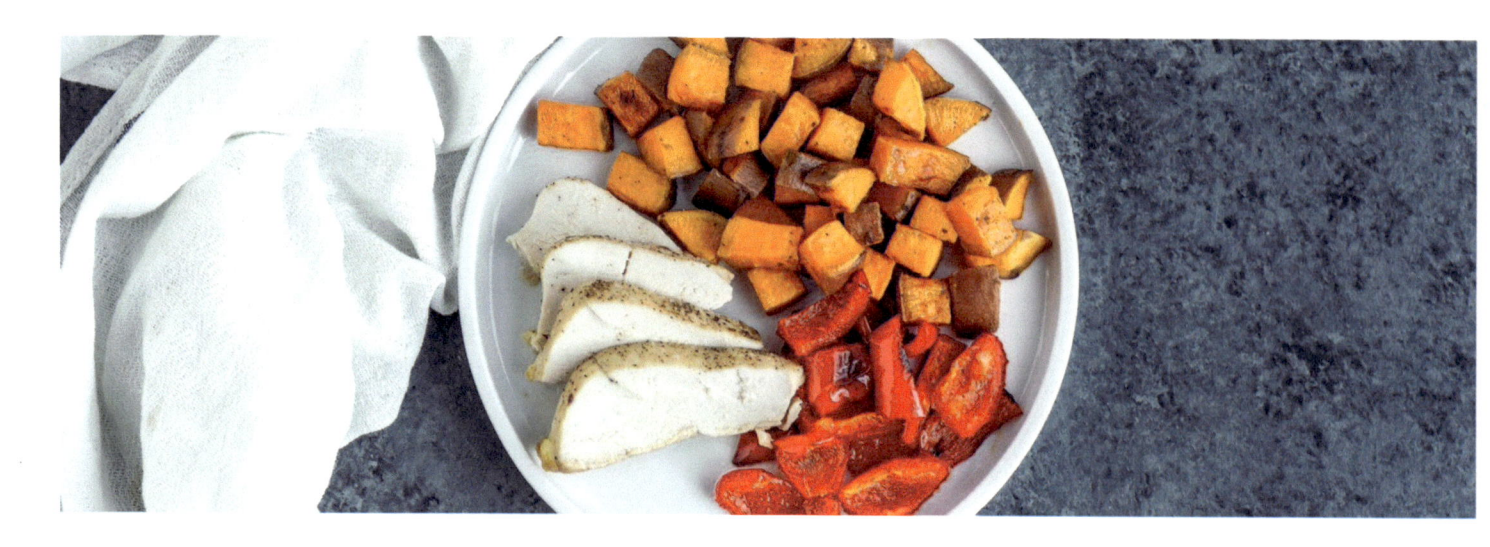

Chicken with Sweet Potato & Peppers

2 servings
35 minutes

Ingredients

10 ozs   Chicken Breast

1   Sweet Potato (large, cut into small cubes)

1   Red Bell Pepper (large, chopped)

1 tbsp   Extra Virgin Olive Oil

        Sea Salt & Black Pepper (to taste)

Directions

1. Preheat oven to 400°F (205°C) and line a large baking sheet with parchment paper.

2. Place the chicken, sweet potato cubes, and bell pepper on the prepared baking sheet. Drizzle with the oil and season with salt and pepper to taste. Toss the sweet potatoes and bell pepper to evenly coat in the seasoning.

3. Bake for about 30 minutes, stirring the potatoes and peppers halfway, or until the chicken is cooked through and vegetables are tender. Allow the chicken to rest for five to 10 minutes before slicing.

4. To serve, season with additional salt and pepper if needed then divide between plates. Enjoy!

Notes

Leftovers: Refrigerate in an airtight container for up to three days.

More Flavor: Add other dried herbs and spices to taste.

No Bell Pepper: Use green beans, zucchini, broccoli, or cauliflower florets.

No Chicken Breast: Use chicken thighs instead.

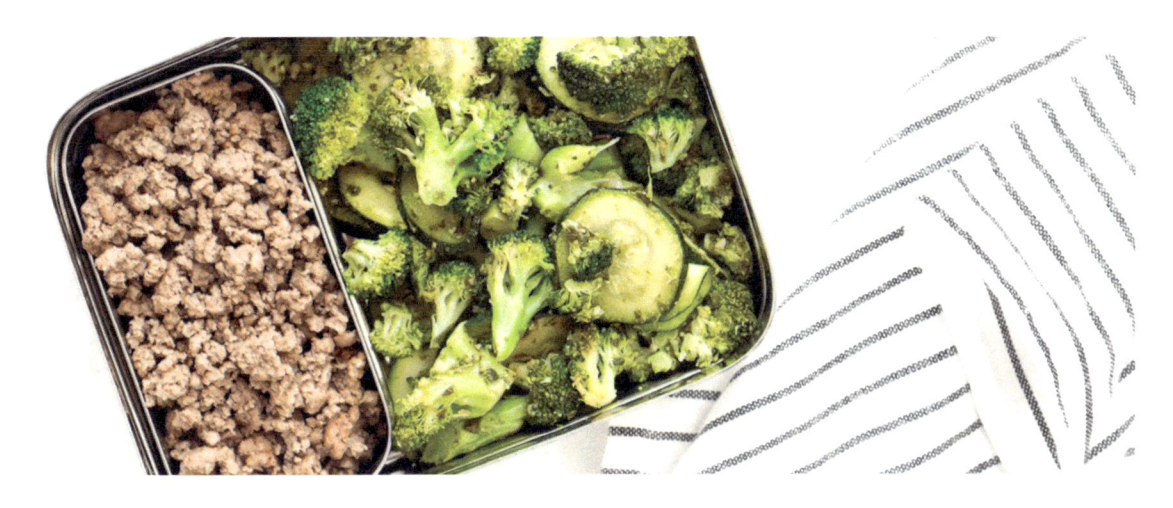

Ground Beef & Pesto Veggies

2 servings
20 minutes

Ingredients

8 ozs	Lean Ground Beef Sea Salt & Black Pepper
1	Zucchini (medium, sliced)
2 cups	Broccoli (chopped into florets)
1 tbsp	Pesto

Directions

1. Heat a nonstick pan over medium heat. Add the beef, salt, and pepper and cook for five to eight minutes, breaking it up as it cooks. Drain extra fat if needed. Set aside.

2. In the same pan over medium heat, add the zucchini slices, broccoli florets, and pesto. Cook until tender, about five to eight minutes.

3. Divide the beef, zucchini, and broccoli into containers. Enjoy!

Notes

Leftovers: Refrigerate in an airtight container for up to three days.

Serving Size: One serving equals approximately four ounces of ground beef, one cup of broccoli, and one cup of zucchini.

More Flavor: Add your choice of herbs and spices.

Additional Toppings: Top with cheese, green onion, yogurt, or salsa.

Make it Vegan: Use crumbled tofu or tempeh instead of ground beef.

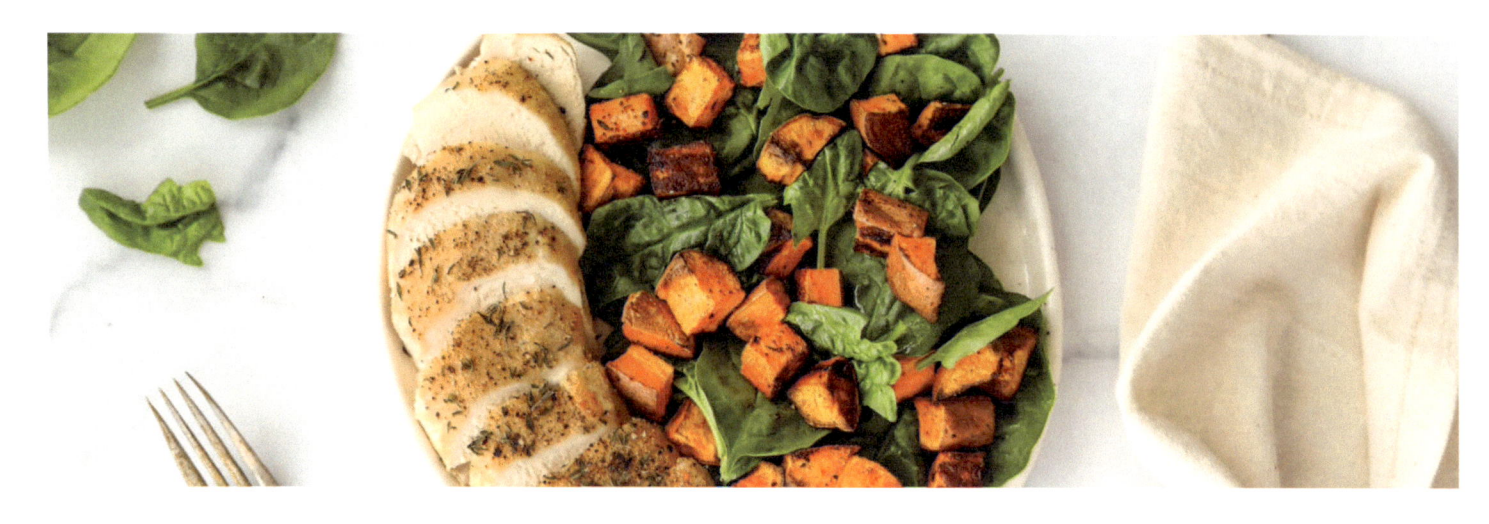

Roasted Chicken & Sweet Potato With Spinach

2 servings
25 minutes

Ingredients

- **1** Sweet Potato (medium, cut into cubes)
- **10 ozs** Chicken Breast (skinless, boneless)
- **1 tsp** Thyme (fresh)
- **1 tsp** Garlic Powder
- **3 cups** Baby Spinach
- Sea Salt & Black Pepper (to taste)

Directions

1. Preheat the oven to 400ºF (205ºC) and line a baking sheet with parchment paper.

2. Place the sweet potatoes and chicken breast on the baking sheet. Season with thyme, garlic powder, salt, and pepper. Bake for 18 to 20 minutes or until the chicken is cooked through and the sweet potatoes are golden.

3. Divide the spinach between plates. Top with the sweet potatoes and chicken. Enjoy!

Notes

Leftovers: Refrigerate in an airtight container in the fridge for up to three days.

More Flavor: Add za'atar and/or paprika to the chicken.

Additional Toppings: Add roasted bell pepper, zucchini, and/or your choice of dressing.

No Fresh Thyme: Use dried thyme or rosemary instead.

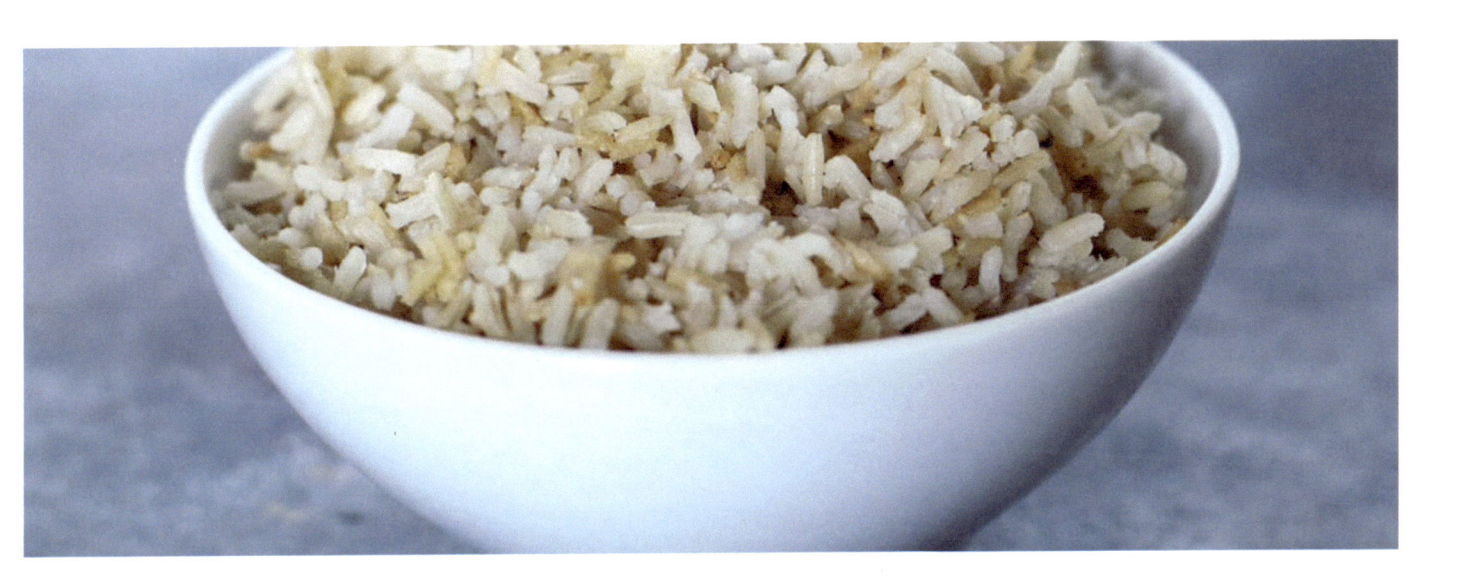

Brown Rice

2 servings
45 minutes

Ingredients

1/2 cup Brown Rice (uncooked)
1 cup Water

Directions

1 Combine the brown rice and water together in a saucepan. Place over high heat and bring to a boil. Once boiling, reduce heat to a simmer and cover with a lid. Let simmer for 40 minutes or until water is absorbed. Remove the lid and fluff with a fork. Enjoy!

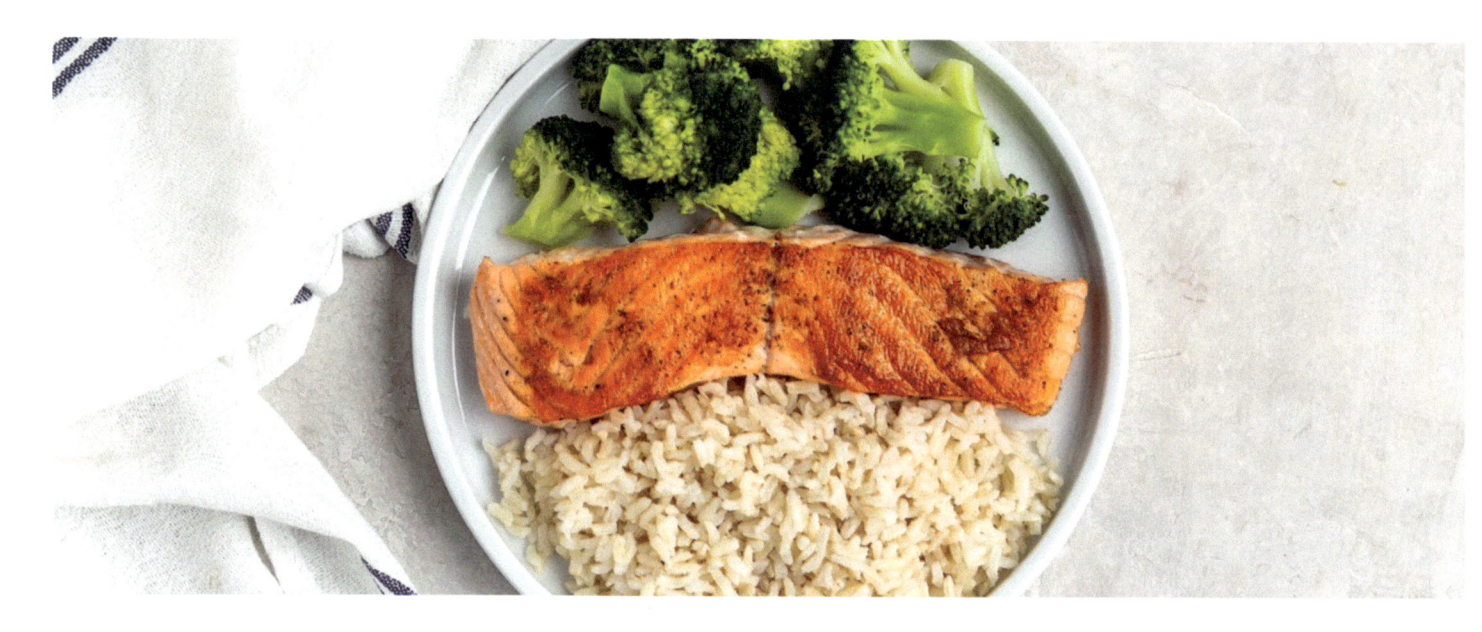

Salmon with Rice & Broccoli

3 servings
30 minutes

Ingredients

3/4 cup   Brown Rice (dry)
1 1/8 lbs   Salmon Fillet
2 1/4 tsps   Extra Virgin Olive Oil
3 cups   Broccoli (cut into florets)
Sea Salt & Black Pepper (to taste)

Directions

1. Cook the rice according to the package directions.

2. Meanwhile, heat the oil in a skillet or cast iron pan over medium heat. Pat the salmon dry with a paper towel and season both sides with salt and pepper to taste. Add the salmon to the pan and cook for four to six minutes per side until cooked through.

3. Meanwhile, steam the broccoli by adding the florets to a steamer basket over boiling water. Cover with a lid and steam for about five minutes, or until tender.

4. To serve, divide the rice, salmon, and broccoli between plates. Enjoy!

Notes

Leftovers: Refrigerate in an airtight container for up to three days.

More Flavor: Season the salmon with dried herbs and spices to taste. Serve with lemon wedges or fresh herbs.

No Brown Rice: Use white rice, jasmine rice, quinoa, cauliflower rice, or couscous.

No Broccoli: Use green beans, cauliflower, or carrots instead.

No Salmon: Use trout, cod, or halibut instead.

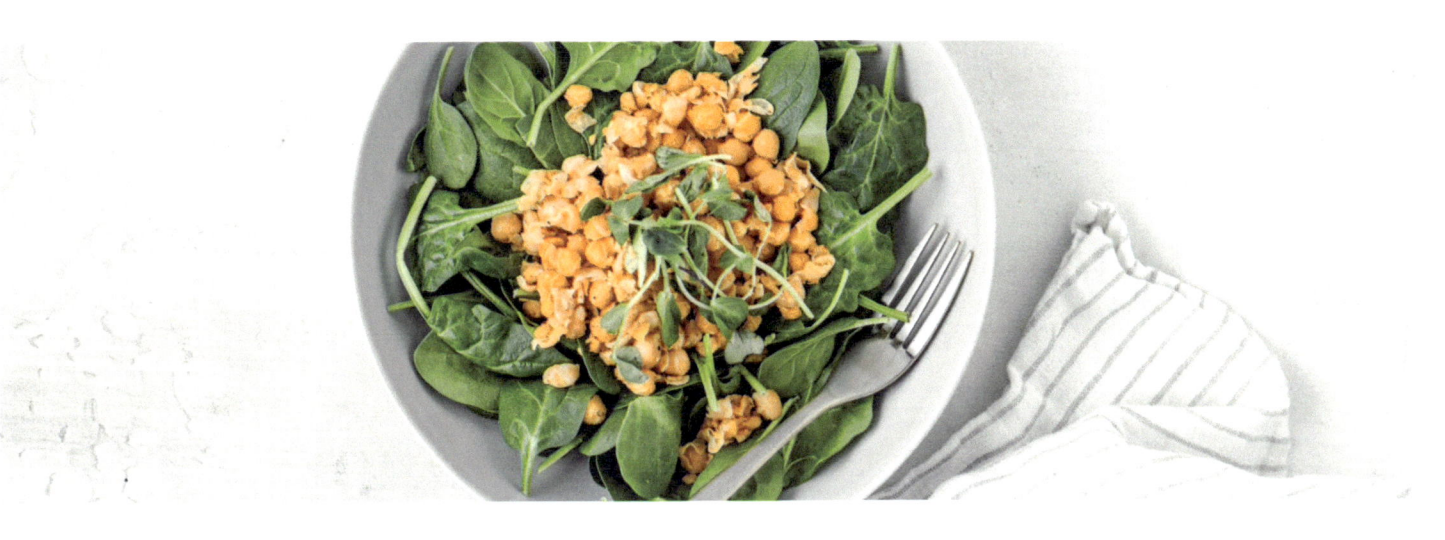

Smashed Chickpea Spinach Salad

2 servings
15 minutes

Ingredients

1 1/2 cups   Chickpeas (cooked, rinsed)
2 tbsps   Extra Virgin Olive Oil (divided)
1   Lemon (large, juiced, divided)
1/2 tsp   Paprika
1   Garlic (clove, minced)
4 cups   Baby Spinach
1/2 cup   Microgreens
Sea Salt & Black Pepper (to taste)

Directions

1. In a bowl, add the chickpeas, half of the oil, half of the lemon juice, paprika, salt, and pepper. Mix to combine. With the back of a fork, lightly mash the chickpeas, leaving some whole.

2. Heat a pan over medium-low heat and add the chickpeas into the pan with the remaining liquid from the bowl. Stir in the minced garlic. Sauté for four to five minutes. Add a splash of water if needed.

3. To assemble, evenly divide the spinach, chickpeas, and microgreens into bowls. Drizzle the remaining oil and lemon juice on top. Season with salt and pepper. Enjoy!

Notes

Leftovers: Refrigerate in an airtight container for up to three days.

More Flavor: Top with your favorite dressing. Sauté the spinach with the chickpeas.

Additional Toppings: Sliced avocado, feta cheese, fresh parsley, dill, cilantro.

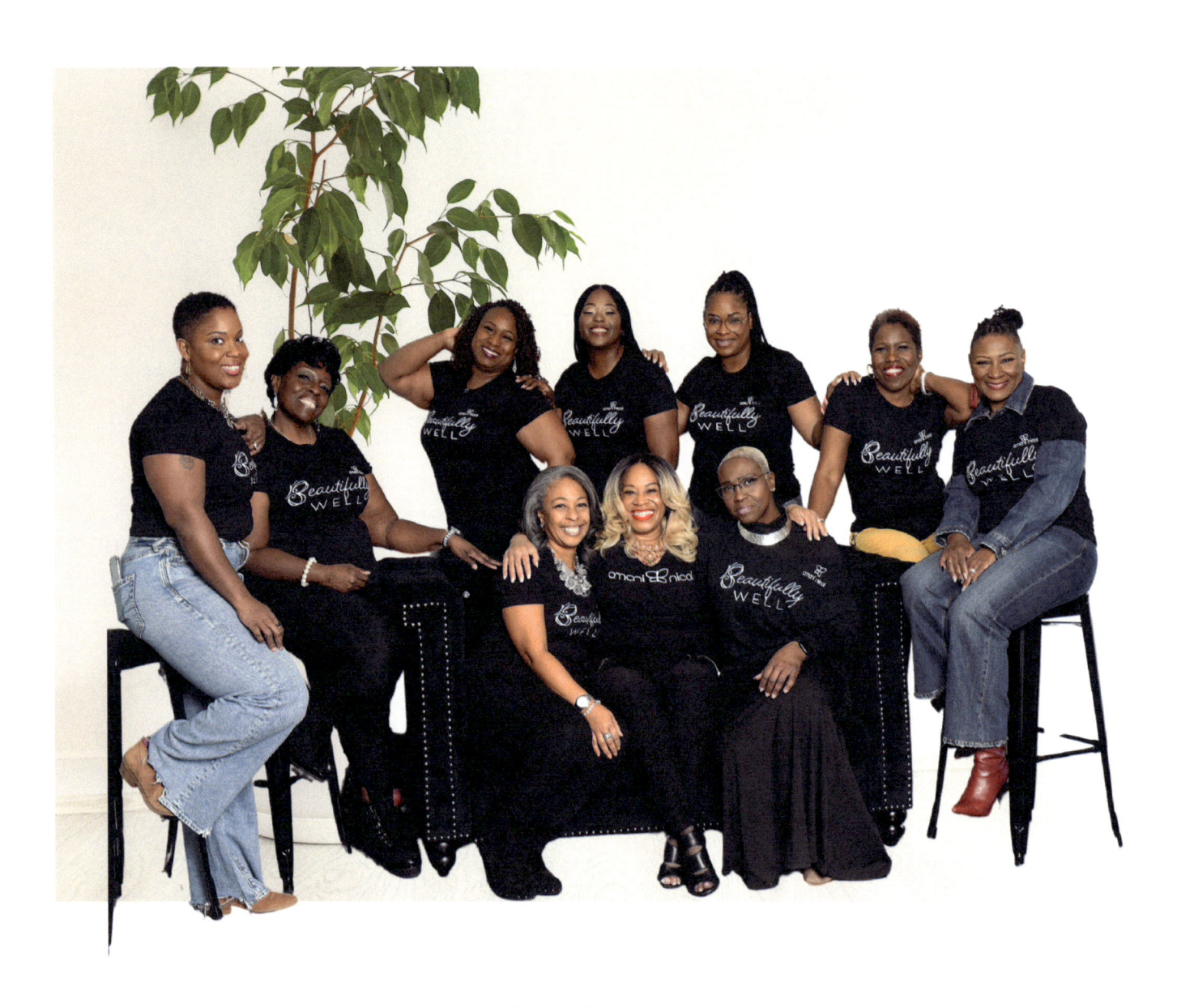

Congratulations Beautiful!

Becoming beautifully well is more than weight loss, it's an investment in you paying dividends now and in the future. What was the biggest takeaway from this journey? What will you continue to do to stay Beautifully Well?

Nik Sweeney

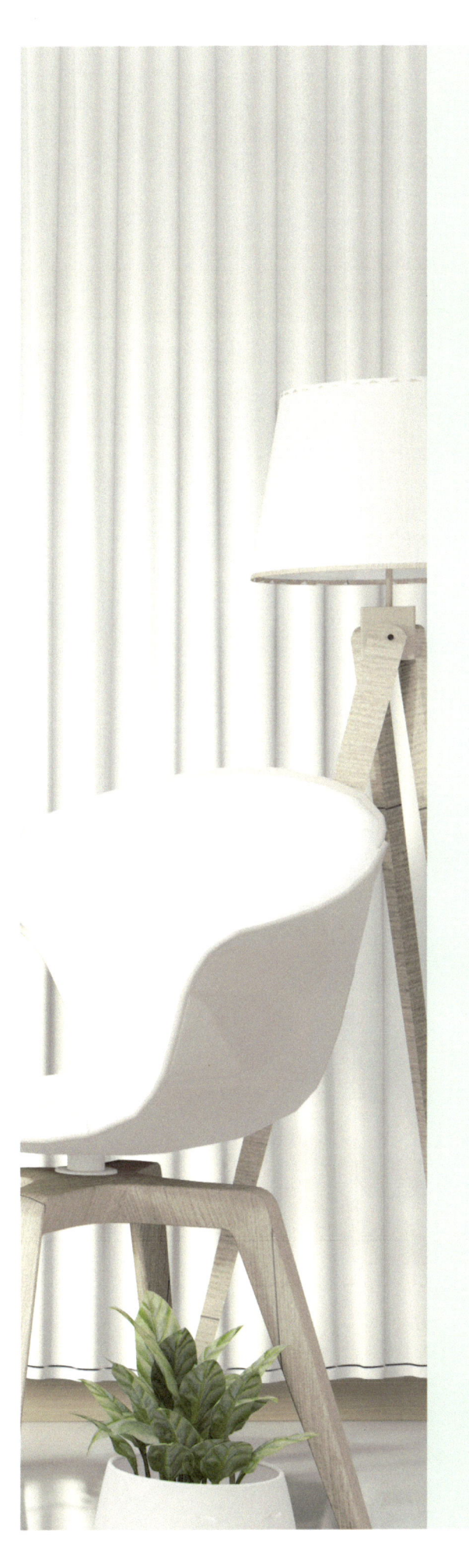

Congratulations Beautiful!

Remember to join our exclusive Facebook Group. *Link inside your digital program.

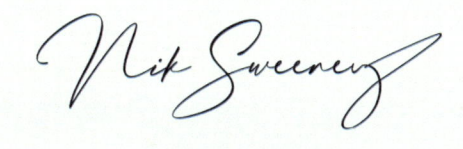

Nik Sweeney

Digital Access Online Program
(scan the QR code)

Amani Nicol Wellness

www.amaninicol.com

info@amaninicol.com

Get social on Instagram & Facebook
@amaninicolwellness

Made in the USA
Columbia, SC
16 February 2025